THE ARITHMETIC OF

DOSAGES AND SOLUTIONS

A Programmed Presentation

The Arithmetic of
Dosages and Solutions

A Programmed Presentation

Laura K. Hart, R.N., B.S.N., M.Ed., M.A., Ph.D.
Associate Professor in Nursing,
University of Iowa College of Nursing,
Iowa City, Iowa

SIXTH EDITION

The C. V. Mosby Company

ST. LOUIS • TORONTO • PRINCETON   1985

MOSBY

A TRADITION OF PUBLISHING EXCELLENCE

Editor: Julie Cardamon
Assistant editor: Bess Arends
Design: Editing, Design, & Production, Inc.
Production: Editing, Design, & Production, Inc.

SIXTH EDITION

Printed in the United States of America

The C.V. Mosby Company
11830 Westline Industrial Drive, St. Louis, Missouri 63146

Library of Congress Cataloging in Publication Data

Hart, Laura K
   The arithmetic of dosages and solutions.

   1. Pharmaceutical arithmetic—Programmed instruction.
2. Drugs—Dosage—Programmed instruction.   3. Nursing—
Programmed instruction.   I. Title.   [DNLM: 1. Drugs—
administration & dosage—programmed texts.   2. Mathematics
—programmed texts.   3. Solutions—programmed texts.
QV 18 H325a]
RS57.H37   1985   615′.14   84-9960
ISBN 0-8016-2089-9

EDP/VH/VH   9   8   7   6   5   4   3   2   1   03/C/325

PREFACE

This text has been compiled primarily to guide student nurses in the study of the arithmetic of dosages and solutions. The technique of programmed instruction used in this text offers students two main advantages: it requires that students become actively involved in the learning process, and it allows them to proceed at their own speed. The programs have been designed so that this course in the arithmetic of dosages and solutions can be completely self-directed. Students are given information in easy-to-digest pieces, a sentence or short paragraph at a time. The information is arranged in logical order, with each step building on the previous one and with the correct answer shown immediately.

The programs were developed on the assumption that all students at the beginning of this course possess the basic mathematical skills of addition, subtraction, multiplication, and division. However, for those who need to brush up on fractions, decimals, percentages, and ratios, a brief review has been included. The programs have been written to ensure that practically all students will get 95% of the answers correct.

In this sixth edition several changes were made to continue and increase the book's usefulness. In the introduction section the arithmetic review has been expanded with the addition of a 56 item arithmetic pretest. The metric unit now includes a discussion of the microgram. In the fractional dosages unit the material discussing insulin has been updated and the practice problem section has been increased. There is a new unit devoted exclusively to the calculation of intravenous flow rates. The appendix has been expanded to include more on the calculation of infants' and children's dosages, and a new practice problem section regarding the calculation of pediatric dosages has been added. These problems were written to serve as a summary for the entire text because they require an understanding of the metric system, household system, fractional dosage, intravenous flow rate calculation, and pediatric dosages. Also throughout the text problems were updated regarding drugs in current use.

Laura K. Hart

CONTENTS

THE ARITHMETIC OF

DOSAGES AND SOLUTIONS

A Programmed Presentation

INTRODUCTION

A BRIEF ARITHMETIC REVIEW

This section has been included for those who need a quick review of the basic rules for fractions, decimals, proportions, and ratios. Because this section is a review, it is not presented in the programmed learning format of the rest of the text. An arithmetic pretest is included to help you practice these skills before attempting to use them in dosage calculations. Examples of how these rules are used to calculate dosages are included in the programmed text where pertinent.

1. **A fraction** is a part of any object, quantity, or digit.

$$
\begin{array}{ll}
1 & \text{numerator} \\
/ & \text{division line} \\
4 & \text{denominator}
\end{array}
$$

2. **To reduce a fraction to its lowest term,** divide the numerator and the denominator by the largest number by which they are both evenly divisible. $\frac{2}{4} = \frac{1}{2}$

3. **To change a mixed number to a fraction,** multiply the denominator by the whole number, add the numerator, and place the sum over the denominator. $3\frac{1}{3} = \frac{10}{3}$

4. **To change an improper fraction to a mixed number,** divide the numerator by the denominator. $\frac{10}{3} = 3\frac{1}{3}$

5. **To add fractions with the same denominator,** add the numerators, write the sum over the common denominator, and reduce the fraction to its lowest term.

$$
\begin{array}{r}
\frac{2}{6} \\
+\frac{2}{6} \\
\hline
\frac{4}{6} = \frac{2}{3}
\end{array}
$$

6. **To add fractions with unlike denominators,** find their lowest common denominator (the lowest number evenly divisible by both denominators). When the numerator and denominator are divided or multiplied by the same number, the value of the fraction remains the same. The numerators are then added and placed over the common denominator.

$$\begin{array}{cc} ^3/_4 & ^3/_4 \\ \underline{+\,^1/_2} = \underline{\,^2/_4} & \text{or} \\ ^5/_4 = 1^1/_4 \end{array} \qquad \begin{array}{cc} 3^3/_4 & 3^3/_4 \\ \underline{+6^1/_2} = \underline{6^2/_4} \\ 9^5/_4 = 10^1/_4 \end{array}$$

7. **To subtract fractions with the same denominator,** find the difference between the numerators and write it over the common denominator. Reduce to lowest terms.

$$\begin{array}{c} ^5/_6 \\ \underline{-\,^2/_6} \\ ^3/_6 = {}^1/_2 \end{array}$$

8. **To subtract fractions with unlike denominators,** find the lowest common denominator, subtract the numerators, and reduce to lowest terms.

$$\begin{array}{cc} ^6/_8 & ^6/_8 \\ \underline{-\,^1/_4} = \underline{\,^2/_8} & \text{or} \\ ^4/_8 = {}^1/_2 \end{array} \qquad \begin{array}{cc} 6^6/_8 & 6^6/_8 \\ \underline{-2^1/_4} = \underline{2^2/_8} \\ 4^4/_8 = 4^1/_2 \end{array}$$

$$\begin{array}{ccc} \text{or} \quad 6^1/_2 & 6^3/_6 & 5^9/_6 \\ \underline{-3^2/_3} = \underline{-3^4/_6} = \underline{-3^4/_6} \\ & & 2^5/_6 \end{array}$$

9. **To multiply fractions,** multiply the numerator by the numerator and the denominator by the denominator. $^1/_2 \times 6 = {}^1/_2 \times {}^6/_1 = {}^6/_2 = 3$

10. **To divide fractions,** invert the divisor and multiply. $^1/_2 \div 6 = {}^1/_2 \div {}^6/_1 = {}^1/_2 \times {}^1/_6 = {}^1/_{12}$

11. **To change a fraction to a decimal,** divide the numerator by the denominator. $^1/_2 = \begin{array}{r} .5 \\ 2\overline{)1.00} \end{array}$

12. **A decimal** refers to ten. Any fraction whose denominator is 10 or a multiple of 10 may be written as a decimal fraction.

Ten millions	Millions	Hundred thousands	Ten thousands	Thousands	Hundreds	Tens	Unit of one	Decimal point	Tenths	Hundredths	Thousandths	Ten thousandths	Hundred thousandths	Millionths	Ten millionths
8	7	6	5	4	3	2	1	·	1	2	3	4	5	6	7

Whole numbers	Decimal numbers

13. **To multiply decimals,** multiply as with whole numbers, but in the product, beginning at the right, point off as many places as there are in the multiplier and the multiplicand combined.

$$
\begin{array}{r}
2.4 \text{ multiplicand} \\
\underline{1.2} \text{ multiplier} \\
48 \\
\underline{24} \\
2.88 \text{ product}
\end{array}
$$

14. **To divide a decimal by a decimal,** move the decimal point of the divisor to the right until the divisor becomes a whole number; then move the decimal point of the dividend the same number of places to the right, adding zeros if necessary.

$$
.002\overline{)4.} = 002.\overline{)4000.}^{\;2000.}
$$

15. **To change a decimal to a fraction,** use the number expressed as the numerator and the number represented by the decimal place as the denominator. $.4 = \frac{4}{10}$ or $.44 = \frac{44}{100}$

16. **To change a decimal to a ratio,** change the decimal to a fraction and then to a ratio. $.4 = \frac{4}{10} = 4:10$ or $2:5$ $.5 = \frac{5}{10} = 5:10$ or $1:2$

17. **A percent** is a fraction whose numerator is expressed and whose denominator is understood to be 100. $20\% = \frac{20}{100}$

18. **To change a percent to a decimal,** remove the percent sign and move the decimal point two places left. $30\% = .30$ $2.5\% = .025$

19. **To change a decimal to a percent,** move the decimal point two places to the right and add the percent sign. $.002 = .2\%$ $.025 = 2.5\%$

20. **To change a percent to a fraction,** divide the percent by 100 and reduce to lowest terms. $50\% = \frac{50}{100} = \frac{1}{2}$ $25\% = \frac{25}{100} = \frac{1}{4}$

21. **To change a percent to a ratio,** use the expressed numerator as the first term and the understood denominator (100) as the second. Reduce to lowest terms. $50\% = 50:100 = 1:2$

22. **To change a ratio to a decimal,** change the ratio to a fraction and then divide the numerator by the denominator. $1:2 = \frac{1}{2} = $
$$
2\overline{)1.00}^{\;.5}
$$

23. **A proportion** shows the relationship between two equal ratios. In a proportion, the product of the means equals the product of the extremes.

3

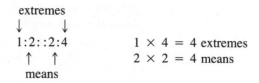

extremes

$$1:2::2:4 \qquad 1 \times 4 = 4 \text{ extremes}$$
$$\qquad\qquad 2 \times 2 = 4 \text{ means}$$

means

If one of the means is unknown, divide the product of the extremes by the known mean.

$$1:?::2:4 \qquad 4 \div 2 = 2$$
$$1 \times 4 = 2 \times ? \qquad 1:2::2:4$$

If one of the extremes is unknown, divide the product of the means by the known extreme.

$$1:2::2:? \qquad 4 \div 1 = 4$$
$$1 \times ? = 2 \times 2 \qquad 1:2::2:4$$

Arithmetic Pretest

A. **Reduce the following to their lowest terms.** (Rule 2)
   1. $8/24$
   2. $10/20$
   3. $4/12$
   4. $5/20$
   5. $25/100$
   6. $50/60$
   7. $14/16$
   8. $12/16$

B. **Convert to improper fractions.** (Rule 3)
   1. $1\frac{6}{8}$
   2. $3\frac{1}{3}$
   3. $6\frac{2}{5}$
   4. $8\frac{1}{6}$
   5. $2\frac{1}{7}$
   6. $3\frac{3}{5}$
   7. $7\frac{1}{3}$
   8. $6\frac{1}{4}$

C. **Convert to mixed numbers.** (Rule 4)
   1. $10/4$
   2. $25/6$
   3. $17/4$
   4. $26/3$
   5. $33/6$
   6. $24/7$
   7. $38/4$
   8. $30/12$

D. **Add and reduce to lowest terms.** (Rule 6)
   1. $\frac{1}{4} + \frac{1}{3}$
   2. $\frac{1}{2} + \frac{2}{3}$
   3. $\frac{3}{4} + \frac{1}{8}$
   4. $\frac{2}{3} + \frac{3}{5}$
   5. $6\frac{1}{4} + 2\frac{1}{5}$
   6. $3\frac{1}{5} + 1\frac{1}{2}$
   7. $5\frac{1}{2} + \frac{1}{6}$
   8. $4\frac{1}{2} + 3\frac{3}{4}$

E. **Subtract and reduce.** (Rule 8)
   1. $\frac{5}{9} - \frac{1}{3}$
   2. $\frac{5}{6} - \frac{2}{3}$
   3. $\frac{2}{3} - \frac{1}{4}$
   4. $\frac{3}{4} - \frac{1}{2}$
   5. $6\frac{1}{4} - 4\frac{1}{8}$
   6. $3\frac{1}{5} - 2\frac{1}{2}$
   7. $4\frac{1}{3} - 1\frac{1}{6}$
   8. $16\frac{2}{3} - 12\frac{1}{2}$

F. **Multiply and reduce.** (Rule 9)
   1. $3 \times \frac{2}{3}$
   2. $25 \times \frac{1}{5}$
   3. $8 \times \frac{3}{4}$
   4. $2 \times \frac{4}{5}$
   5. $\frac{2}{3} \times \frac{5}{10}$
   6. $\frac{1}{4} \times \frac{4}{5}$
   7. $3\frac{2}{3} \times 2\frac{5}{6}$
   8. $2\frac{5}{6} \times 1\frac{3}{5}$

G. **Divide and reduce.** (Rule 10)
   1. $\frac{4}{5} \div \frac{3}{4}$
   2. $\frac{3}{5} \div \frac{1}{3}$
   3. $\frac{1}{4} \div \frac{1}{2}$
   4. $\frac{1}{2} \div \frac{1}{4}$
   5. $2 \div \frac{4}{5}$
   6. $5 \div \frac{3}{4}$
   7. $2\frac{2}{3} \div 1\frac{1}{4}$
   8. $\frac{2}{5} \div 2\frac{1}{4}$

H. **Express the following percentages as common fractions, decimals, and ratios.**

	Percent	Common fraction (Use Rule 20)	Decimal (Use Rule 18)	Ratio (Use Rule 21)
1.	2%			
2.	10%			
3.	5%			
4.	50%			
5.	25%			
6.	200%			
7.	30%			
8.	16%			
		(Use Rules 20 and 10)	(Use Rules 11 and 18)	
9.	⅕%			
10.	¼%			
		(Use Rules 3, 20, and 10)	(Use Rules 3, 11, and 18)	
11.	12½%			
12.	6¼%			

I. **Compute the following means and extremes.** (Rule 23)

1. $5:20::10:?$ 5. $6:?::5:20$
2. $3:9::6:?$ 6. $2:8::?:20$
3. $?:4::5:10$ 7. $5:6::?:12$
4. $?:12::3:4$ 8. $4:8::?:15$

J. **Compute the following, using Rule 23.**

1. If property is taxed at $200 per $10,000, what is the tax on a house assessed at $70,000?
2. If there are 48 pieces of candy in 2 pounds, how many are there in 3½ pounds?
3. If there are 22 cookies in 4 boxes, how many are there in 6 boxes?
4. If a car traveled 75 miles in 3 hours, how far would it travel in 8 hours moving at the same rate?

Arithmetic Pretest Answers

A.
1. $\frac{1}{3}$
2. $\frac{1}{2}$
3. $\frac{1}{3}$
4. $\frac{1}{4}$
5. $\frac{1}{4}$
6. $\frac{5}{6}$
7. $\frac{7}{8}$
8. $\frac{3}{4}$

B.
1. $\frac{14}{8}$
2. $\frac{10}{3}$
3. $\frac{32}{5}$
4. $\frac{49}{6}$
5. $\frac{15}{7}$
6. $\frac{18}{5}$
7. $\frac{22}{3}$
8. $\frac{25}{4}$

C.
1. $2\frac{1}{2}$
2. $4\frac{1}{6}$
3. $4\frac{1}{4}$
4. $8\frac{2}{3}$
5. $5\frac{1}{2}$
6. $3\frac{3}{7}$
7. $9\frac{1}{2}$
8. $2\frac{1}{2}$

D.
1. $\frac{1}{4} + \frac{1}{3} = \frac{3}{12} + \frac{4}{12} = \frac{7}{12}$
2. $\frac{1}{2} + \frac{2}{3} = \frac{3}{6} + \frac{4}{6} = \frac{7}{6} = 1\frac{1}{6}$
3. $\frac{3}{4} + \frac{1}{8} = \frac{6}{8} + \frac{1}{8} = \frac{7}{8}$
4. $\frac{2}{3} + \frac{3}{5} = \frac{10}{15} + \frac{9}{15} = \frac{19}{15} = 1\frac{4}{15}$
5. $6\frac{1}{4} + 2\frac{1}{5} = 6\frac{5}{20} + 2\frac{4}{20} = 8\frac{9}{20}$
6. $3\frac{1}{5} + 1\frac{1}{2} = 3\frac{2}{10} + 1\frac{5}{10} = 4\frac{7}{10}$
7. $5\frac{1}{2} + \frac{1}{6} = 5\frac{3}{6} + \frac{1}{6} = 5\frac{4}{6} = 5\frac{2}{3}$
8. $4\frac{1}{2} + 3\frac{3}{4} = 4\frac{2}{4} + 3\frac{3}{4} = 7\frac{5}{4} = 8\frac{1}{4}$

E.
1. $\frac{5}{9} - \frac{1}{3} = \frac{5}{9} - \frac{3}{9} = \frac{2}{9}$
2. $\frac{5}{6} - \frac{2}{3} = \frac{5}{6} - \frac{4}{6} = \frac{1}{6}$
3. $\frac{2}{3} - \frac{1}{4} = \frac{8}{12} - \frac{3}{12} = \frac{5}{12}$
4. $\frac{3}{4} - \frac{1}{2} = \frac{3}{4} - \frac{2}{4} = \frac{1}{4}$
5. $6\frac{1}{4} - 4\frac{1}{8} = 6\frac{2}{8} - 4\frac{1}{8} = 2\frac{1}{8}$
6. $3\frac{1}{5} - 2\frac{1}{2} = 3\frac{2}{10} - 2\frac{5}{10} = 2\frac{12}{10} - 2\frac{5}{10} = \frac{7}{10}$
7. $4\frac{1}{3} - 1\frac{1}{6} = 4\frac{2}{6} - 1\frac{1}{6} = 3\frac{1}{6}$
8. $16\frac{2}{3} - 12\frac{1}{2} = 16\frac{4}{6} - 12\frac{3}{6} = 4\frac{1}{6}$

F.
1. $3 \times \frac{2}{3} = \frac{3}{1} \times \frac{2}{3} = \frac{6}{3} = 2$
2. $25 \times \frac{1}{5} = \frac{25}{1} \times \frac{1}{5} = \frac{25}{5} = 5$
3. $8 \times \frac{3}{4} = \frac{8}{1} \times \frac{3}{4} = \frac{24}{4} = 6$
4. $2 \times \frac{4}{5} = \frac{2}{1} \times \frac{4}{5} = \frac{8}{5} = 1\frac{3}{5}$
5. $\frac{2}{3} \times \frac{5}{10} = \frac{10}{30} = \frac{1}{3}$
6. $\frac{1}{4} \times \frac{4}{5} = \frac{4}{20} = \frac{1}{5}$
7. $3\frac{2}{3} \times 2\frac{5}{6} = \frac{11}{3} \times \frac{17}{6} = \frac{187}{18} = 10\frac{7}{18}$
8. $2\frac{5}{6} \times 1\frac{3}{5} = \frac{17}{6} \times \frac{8}{5} = \frac{136}{30} = 4\frac{16}{30} = 4\frac{8}{15}$

G. 1. $\frac{4}{5} \div \frac{3}{4} = \frac{4}{5} \times \frac{4}{3} = \frac{16}{15} = 1\frac{1}{15}$
    2. $\frac{3}{5} \div \frac{1}{3} = \frac{3}{5} \times \frac{3}{1} = \frac{9}{5} = 1\frac{4}{5}$
    3. $\frac{1}{4} \div \frac{1}{2} = \frac{1}{4} \times \frac{2}{1} = \frac{2}{4} = \frac{1}{2}$
    4. $\frac{1}{2} \div \frac{1}{4} = \frac{1}{2} \times \frac{4}{1} = \frac{4}{2} = 2$
    5. $2 \div \frac{4}{5} = \frac{2}{1} \times \frac{5}{4} = \frac{10}{4} = 2\frac{2}{4} = 2\frac{1}{2}$
    6. $5 \div \frac{3}{4} = \frac{5}{1} \times \frac{4}{3} = \frac{20}{3} = 6\frac{2}{3}$
    7. $2\frac{2}{3} \div 1\frac{1}{4} = \frac{8}{3} \times \frac{4}{5} = \frac{32}{15} = 2\frac{2}{15}$
    8. $\frac{2}{5} \div 2\frac{1}{4} = \frac{2}{5} \times \frac{4}{9} = \frac{8}{45}$

		Common fraction	Decimal	Ratio
H.		(See Rule 20)	(See Rule 18)	(See Rule 21)
	1.	$\frac{2}{100}$ or $\frac{1}{50}$	.02	2:100 or 1:50
	2.	$\frac{10}{100}$ or $\frac{1}{10}$	.1	10:100 or 1:10
	3.	$\frac{5}{100}$ or $\frac{1}{20}$	.05	5:100 or 1:20
	4.	$\frac{50}{100}$ or $\frac{1}{2}$	.5	50:100 or 1:2
	5.	$\frac{25}{100}$ or $\frac{1}{4}$	.25	25:100 or 1:4
	6.	$\frac{200}{100}$ or 2	2.0	200:100 or 2:1
	7.	$\frac{30}{100}$ or $\frac{3}{10}$	.3	30:100 or 3:10
	8.	$\frac{16}{100}$ or $\frac{4}{25}$	.16	16:100 or 4:25
		(See Rules 20 and 10)	(See Rules 11 and 18)	
	9.	$\frac{1}{500}$	.2% = .002	1:500
	10.	$\frac{1}{400}$	.25% = .0025	1:400
		(See Rules 3, 20, and 10)	(See Rules 3, 11, and 18)	
	11.	$\frac{1}{8}$	.125	1:8
	12.	$\frac{1}{16}$	.0625	1:16

I. 1. $5x = 200$
        $x = 40$
    2. $3x = 54$
        $x = 18$
    3. $10x = 20$
        $x = 2$
    4. $4x = 36$
        $x = 9$
    5. $5x = 120$
        $x = 24$
    6. $8x = 40$
        $x = 5$
    7. $6x = 60$
        $x = 10$
    8. $8x = 60$
        $x = 7.5$

J. 1. $10,000:200::70,000:x$
        $10,000x = 14,000,000$
        $x = 1400$
    4. $75:3::x:8$
        $3x = 600$
        $x = 200$
    2. $48:2::x:3.5$
        $2x = 168$
        $x = 84$
    3. $22:4::x:6$
        $4x = 132$
        $x = 33$

ABBREVIATIONS COMMONLY USED IN MEDICATION ORDERS

aa	of each (equal parts)	PO	by mouth
ac	before meals	PR	by rectum
AD	right ear	prn	when required
ad lib	as much as desired	q	every
Aq	water	qd	every day
AS or AL	left ear	qh	every hour
AU	both ears	q2h	every two hours
bid	twice a day	q3h	every three hours
c̄	with	q4h	every four hours
cap	capsules	qid	four times a day
dil	dilute	qod	every other day
fl	fluid	s̄	without
h	hour	ss	a half
hs	hours of sleep (bedtime)	Sol	solution
IM	intramuscular	Stat	immediately
IV	intravenous	SQ, SC, or H	subcutaneous
OD	right eye	supp	suppository
OS or OL	left eye	tab	tablet
os	mouth	tid	three times a day
OU	both eyes	tr or tinct	tincture
pc	after meals	ung	ointment
per	by		

METRIC SYSTEM

In order to administer medications accurately, a nurse must understand the systems used for weighing and measuring drugs. During the past 10 years, use of the metric system for weighing and measuring drugs has increased rapidly. Efforts to have the metric system used exclusively are intensifying. However, a number of places in the United States still make limited use of the apothecaries' system. For this reason, a nurse must still understand both systems and how they may be interchanged.

1. The metric system, which employs the decimal scale, is composed of units measuring *length, volume,* and *weight.* Because the metric system employs the decimal scale, is its numerical scale based on units of 4, 10, or 22? _____

    10

2. Before considering the metric system's three units of measure, those of length, volume, and _____, let us first examine the use of the decimal scale in the metric system.

    weight

3. A prefix (the first syllable or part of a word) is used to modify word's meaning. The prefixes attached to metric designations of length, volume, and weight indicate the unit of 10 that applies to that metric measure. The words used to designate a metric measure identify both the type of measure being used (length, _____, or weight), and the multiple of _____ that applies to that measure in the given situation.

    volume
    10

4. The numerical scale of the metric system is divided into six units of 10. Because the prefixes attached to metric measures indicate which unit of 10 applies, only _____ prefixes are needed to modify metric measures.

    6

5. Three of the six prefixes indicate multiples of 10, and three indicate fractional units. The prefixes indicating multiples of 10 are deka, designating units of 10; hecto, designating units of 100; and kilo, designating units of 1000. A _____ of a unit would be 100 times larger than a deka.

    kilo

6. Of the three prefixes used to indicate multiples of 10, the one most frequently used by the nurse is the prefix that refers to 1000 units. This prefix is _____.

    kilo

1000	**7.** Kilo is used in the word kiloliter to indicate a quantity _____ liters in volume.
1000	**8.** Kilo is used in the word kilometer to indicate a distance _____ meters in length.
kilogram	**9.** The quantity of 1000 grams in weight is usually referred to as a _____.
kilo	**10.** The three prefixes that indicate the multiples of units are of Greek derivation. Of these prefixes, the nurse most frequently uses the prefix _____.
fractions or divisions	**11.** The prefixes that indicate the divisions or *fractions* of a unit are of Latin derivation. Prefixes are used to indicate not only multiples of a unit but _____ of a unit of measure as well.
10	**12.** Because the metric system uses the decimal scale, fractional parts of metric units are always indicated with decimal numbers. The three prefixes that indicate the divisions of the metric units are deci, referring to .1 of a unit; centi, referring to .01 of a unit; and milli, referring to .001 of a unit. Each is a division of _____.
smaller	**13.** The divisional prefix of deci, referring to .1, is infrequently used in medical measurements. The prefix centi, referring to .01 of a unit, indicates a *(smaller? larger?)* portion of the unit than the prefix deci.
.001	**14.** Deci indicates a unit 10 times larger than does centi. A centi of a unit is 10 times larger than a milli. Therefore, if a deci equals .1 of a unit and a centi equals .01 of a unit, then a milli equals _____ of a unit.
centi milli	**15.** The divisional prefixes most commonly used in hospital terminology are the centi and the milli. The prefix _____ refers to .01 of a unit and _____ refers to .001 of a unit.
1000 .01 .001	**16.** Of the six prefixes used to indicate multiples or fractions of a unit, only three are used with frequency in the hospital. The prefix kilo is used to indicate _____ times the unit; the prefix centi is used to indicate _____ part of a unit; and the prefix milli is used to indicate _____ part of a unit.
centi; milli kilo	**17.** Identify the prefix that indicates the following multiples or divisions of a metric unit: _____, .01 unit; _____, .001 unit; _____, 1000 units.
meter	**18.** The *meter* is the fundamental unit of the metric system. It is called the fundamental unit because it is from this standard of linear measure that the other two metric units of weight and volume are derived. As the name implies, the _____ is the fundamental unit of the metric system.
	19. An example of the use of this linear measure is the calibration of the sphygmomanometer, an instrument used to measure the blood

pressure. Its scale is calibrated in millimeters. This indicates that each division of length represents .001 of a _____.

meter

20. When very small or precise measurements are needed, the millimeter is used. However, for larger measures, such as the length of a newborn infant, the centimeter is the unit used. The centimeter (cm) is _____ times larger than the millimeter (mm). Note the abbreviations.

10

21. Height is often measured in cm. A cm is ⅖ or .3937 parts of an inch. You can determine how tall a person is in cm by using the proportion rule. (See pp. 3 and 4 for an explanation of how to solve a proportion problem.) A person who is 60 inches tall is also _____ cm tall.

152

$$\frac{1 \text{ cm}}{.3937 \text{ in}} :: \frac{? \text{ cm}}{60 \text{ in}}$$

Cross multiply: $.3937x = 60$

$$3937\overline{)600000.}^{152.4}$$

$$x = 152 \text{ cm}$$

22. A 51-cm infant is _____ inches long.

20

$$\frac{1 \text{ cm}}{.3937 \text{ in}} :: \frac{51 \text{ cm}}{? \text{ in}}$$

23. A centimeter is *(larger? smaller?)* than an inch.

smaller

24. The metric unit of capacity or volume is the *liter* (L). It was decided that the volume of a liter should be that which could be contained in a cube measuring exactly 1 decimeter (dm) in length on all sides. This is how the standard for the metric unit of volume, the _____, was derived from the fundamental linear unit, the _____.

liter
meter

25. The prefix deci means .1; therefore, a decimeter equals _____ of a meter.

.1

26. If a centimeter is .01 meter and a decimeter is .1 meter, then there are _____ cm in 1 dm.

10

27. If 10 cm equal 1 dm, and if a cube measuring 1 dm on all sides contains 1 L, then a cube measuring 10 cm on all sides would also hold the volume of a _____.

liter

28. If you take the side measurement of a 10-cm container and cube it (take it to the third power), you will have the answer to how many cubes measuring a cm on all sides can be held in a liter volume. You can cube 10 cm in the following manner:

$$\frac{\text{1st power 2nd power}}{(10 \text{ cm}) \times (10 \text{ cm})} = 100 \text{ cm} \times \frac{\text{3rd power}}{(10 \text{ cm})} = \frac{1000}{\text{cubic cm}}$$

To determine total volume, the side measures are taken to the third power because a cube is three dimensional. Therefore, 1000 cubes measuring 1 cm on all sides exactly fill the capacity of a _____.

liter

1000

29. If 1000 cm cubes equal a liter, then a liter contains _____ cubic centimeters (cc).

30. As you recall, the prefix milli indicates .001 parts of a unit. Therefore, a milliliter is what part of a liter? _____

.001

31. The milliliter is the division of a liter that is most commonly used in the hospital, and it is abbreviated ml. Beeause a milliliter is .001 of a liter, there are _____ ml in a liter.

1000

32. If there are 1000 ml in a liter and 1000 cc in a liter, then 1 cc could contain _____ ml of material.

1

33. 1 L = _____ ml; 1 L = _____ cc; 1 ml = _____ cc.

1000; 1000; 1

34. It is important to know this relationship between the volume and capacity measures in the metric system because liquid drugs are usually ordered in relation to their volume but are measured according to the cc capacity of the container in which they will be distributed. Note the markings on the 2-cc syringe below.

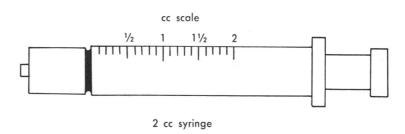

2 cc syringe

If a patient is to receive an injection of 1.5 ml of a medication, this volume should be measured by filling a syringe to the _____ cc marking.

1.5

35. Note that medicine glasses are also marked according to their cc capacity. As in the example on p. 14, some are marked with both the cc capacity scale and the ml volume scale. If you administer 15 ml of a medication, the medicine glass should be filled to the _____ cc marking.

15

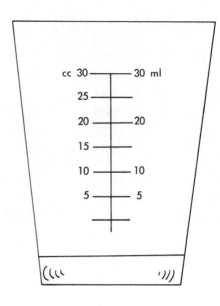

36. Usually in the hospital, fractional parts of a liter are expressed in milliliters. For example, a pitcher containing ½ L of fluid contains 500 ml of fluid. If a glass contained ¼ L of water, how many milliliters would it contain? _____

250

37. Multiples of liters are also usually expressed in milliliters. For example, 1½ L of fluid would be referred to as 1500 ml of fluid. What is the amount of 1¾ L of fluid expressed in milliliters? _____

1750 ml

38. In the hospital, fluid volumes are usually expressed in milliliters; however, it is necessary to know that 1 ml = _____ cc because syringe and medicine-glass capacities are frequently expressed in cubic centimeters.

1

39. A syringe filled to a 2-cc capacity contains _____ ml of drug, and a medicine glass filled to a 30-cc capacity contains _____ ml of drug.

2

30

40. Using these two previously established standards, the meter and the liter, the original standard unit of weight was established. It was decided that a kilogram would be the weight of a liter of distilled water weighed at 4°C and 760 mm of pressure. The temperature had to be held constant because fluid will expand and contract with a change in temperature. The original standard unit of weight, the _____, weighs approximately 2.2 pounds (lbs).

kilogram

2.2

41. The kilogram, weighing approximately _____ lbs, is frequently used in hospitals to express body weights.

80	**42.** A person weighing 176 pounds weighs _____ kilograms (Kg):

$$\frac{2.2 \text{ lbs}}{1 \text{ Kg}} :: \frac{176 \text{ lbs}}{? \text{ Kg}}$$

43. A person weighing 60 Kg weighs _____ pounds.

132

44. The kilogram proved to be too large to meet the practical needs of pharmacists, so they decided to use the gram as their basic metric unit of weight. If the kilogram is 1000 grams, then the basic unit of weight, the gram, is _____ of a kilogram.

.001

45. Fractional parts of a gram are usually expressed in milligrams. As you remember, milli means _____ of a unit; so a milligram is _____ of a gram (g).

.001
.001

46. The milligram (mg), .001 of a gram, is as frequently used to express drug weights as is the gram. Because the milligram is _____ times smaller than the gram, it is very easy to change grams to milligrams. Simply multiply the number of grams by 1000, or move the decimal point three places to the right. For example: 1 g = 1000 mg; .5 g = 500 mg; .1 g = _____ mg.

1000

100

47. Convert the following to milligrams.

900 mg
3 mg
70 mg

   .9 g = _____
.003 g = _____
 .07 g = _____

48. To change milligrams to grams, the process is simply reversed. The number of milligrams is divided by 1000, or the decimal point is moved three places to the left. For example: 600 mg = .6 g; 200 mg = _____ g

.2

49. Convert the following to grams.

.4 g
.08 g
1.5 g

  400 mg = _____
   80 mg = _____
1500 mg = _____

50. In the metric system, the basic units of length, volume, and weight are the _____, _____, and _____ (same sequence).

meter; liter; gram

51. The meter is a unit of _____. The height of patients is usually recorded in the measure of _____ (.01 meter).

length
centimeter

52. The liter is a unit of _____. Fluid volumes are usually expressed in _____ (ml).

volume
milliliters

53. 1 ml = _____ cc. The capacities of syringes and medicine glasses are often expressed in both _____ and _____.

1
ml; cc

54. The kilogram is the original standard unit of _____. However, the _____ is used as the basic metric unit of weight.

weight
gram

kilograms
grams
milligrams

55. The weight of patients is usually recorded in _____.

56. Drug weights are usually expressed in _____ (g) or _____ (mg).

57. Convert the following:

.4
5000
500
.002
1.3

$$400 \text{ mg} = \text{_____} \text{ g}$$
$$5 \text{ g} = \text{_____} \text{ mg}$$
$$.5 \text{ g} = \text{_____} \text{ mg}$$
$$2 \text{ mg} = \text{_____} \text{ g}$$
$$1300 \text{ mg} = \text{_____} \text{ g}$$

58. In some instances, such as with hormones, the dosage required is so small that even the measure of mg is too large. The measure used for these situations is called a microgram (mcg or µg). This Greek-derived prefix means small and is used to designate an amount one-millionth (10^{-6}) the size of the basic unit. An mcg = .000001 _____.

gram
.001
1000

59. If 1 mcg = .000001 g, then 1 mcg = _____ mg.

60. Because the mg is _____ times larger than the mcg, it is essential that these measures not be confused. Unfortunately, the abbreviation mcg looks very much like mg.

.001

61. Weight is the only unit of measure for which the nurse commonly uses the division of micro. The microgram (mcg) = _____ mg.

62. Identify the following abbreviations:

milliliter; centimeter
cubic centimeter; kilogram
milligram; liter
gram; microgram
microgram

ml _____   cm _____
cc _____   Kg _____
mg _____   L _____
g _____   mcg _____
µg _____

mg

63. When administering medications you will find drug dosages expressed in the weight measures of g, _____, or mcg.

64. Convert the following:

300
.5
.5
200
3.5
10

$$.3 \text{ mg} = \text{_____} \text{ mcg}$$
$$500 \text{ mcg} = \text{_____} \text{ mg}$$
$$500 \text{ mg} = \text{_____} \text{ g}$$
$$.2 \text{ g} = \text{_____} \text{ mg}$$
$$3500 \text{ mg} = \text{_____} \text{ g}$$
$$.01 \text{ mg} = \text{_____} \text{ mcg}$$

65. When administering medications, if you have a choice of tablets of various dosage amounts, always try to administer the least possible number of tablets or capsules out of convenience for the patient and for economy. If the doctor orders 1 g of a drug to be administered and you have tablets of 250 mg and 500 mg, you should give two 500-mg tablets because you always try to give the _____ number of tablets possible.

66. If you had only 250-mg tablets available, how many tablets should you give to fill the doctor's order of 1 g? _____

67. The doctor orders 5 mg of a drug to be given, and 1-mg tablets, 2-mg tablets, and 2.5-mg tablets are available. What should you give?
_____

68. If the doctor orders 250 mg of a drug to be given and you have 50-mg, 100-mg and 200-mg capsules available, what should you give?
_____
_____.

69. Many tablets, such as layered tablets or sustained-action tablets, do not have the drug equally distributed throughout the tablet. Therefore, when you are preparing drugs for oral administration, you should never break a tablet for a fractional dose unless the tablet is scored. A scored tablet has a dividing line exactly through its center, and each half of the tablet supposedly contains the same amount of the drug. You cannot be sure that both sides of the tablet contain an equal amount of the drug unless the tablet is _____, nor can you be sure that you will be able to break a tablet in equal halves.

70. Because capsules are gelatin cylinders containing powders, oils, or liquids, the only solid drug form that should ever be divided by the nurse for a fractional dose is a _____ tablet. However, because there is never an absolute surety about equal distribution of drugs throughout any tablet, it is best never to split tablets if another, more accurate, method of administration is available.

Review of Metric System Equivalents

Linear measure:	1 meter	=	10 decimeters (dm)
	1 meter	=	100 centimeters (cm)
			(1 cm = .3937 inches)
	1 meter	=	1000 millimeters (mm)
	10 meters	=	1 dekameter (Dm)
	100 meters	=	1 hectometer (Hm)
	1000 meters	=	1 kilometer (Km) (⅝ mile)

Volume:	1 liter (L)	=	10 deciliters (dl)
	1 liter	=	100 centiliters (cl)
	1 liter	=	1000 milliliters (ml)
	10 liters	=	1 dekaliter (Dl)
	100 liters	=	1 hectoliter (Hl)
	1000 liters	=	1 kiloliter (Kl)

Weight:	1 gram (g)	=	10 decigrams (dg)
	1 gram	=	100 centigrams (cg)
	1 gram	=	1000 milligrams (mg)
	10 grams	=	1 deckagram (Dg)
	100 grams	=	1 hectogram (Hg)
	1000 grams	=	1 kilogram (Kg) (2.2 lbs)
	.000001 gram or		
	.001 milligram	=	1 microgram (mcg or μg)

Metric System Practice Problems

1. 1 L = _____ cc
2. 1 L = _____ ml
3. 500 cc = _____ L
4. 1 cm = _____ mm
5. 5 cm = _____ mm
6. 0.2 cm = _____ mm
7. 5 mm = _____ cm
8. 0.5 mm = _____ cm
9. 1 g = _____ mg
10. 0.5 g = _____ mg
11. 0.3 g = _____ mg
12. 0.015 g = _____ mg
13. 0.008 g = _____ mg
14. 8 mg = _____ g
15. 10 mg = _____ g
16. 5 mg = _____ g
17. 15 mg = _____ g
18. 30 mg = _____ g
19. 60 mg = _____ g
20. 1 mg = _____ g
21. 0.2 mg = _____ g

22. 0.2 mg = _____ mcg
23. 0.5 mg = _____ g
24. 0.04 mg = _____ g
25. 0.04 mg = _____ mcg
26. 1.2 g = _____ mg
27. 0.0004 g = _____ mg
28. 0.5 L = _____ ml
29. 50 g = _____ Kg
30. 0.002 g = _____ mg
31. 20 cc = _____ ml
32. 5 ml = _____ cc
33. 50 Kg = _____ lbs
34. 4000 g = _____ Kg
35. 4000 g = _____ lbs
36. 50 lbs = _____ Kg
37. 120 lbs = _____ Kg
38. 50 mg = _____ g
39. 0.005 g = _____ mg
40. 80 cm = _____ inches
41. 1 mcg = _____ mg
42. .006 mg = _____ mcg

43. You are to give 0.650 g of aspirin. The label reads, "Aspirin 325 mg." How many tablets should you give? _____

44. You are to give 2 g of Gantanol. The label reads, "Gantanol 500 mg." How many tablets should you give? _____

45. You are to order from the pharmacy enough medication to fill the order Benadryl 50 mg, bid × 3 days. Benadryl is available from the pharmacy in 25-mg capsules. How many capsules should you order for the 3 days? _____

46. Erythromycin is available in 250-mg capsules. The doctor orders erythromycin 250 mg, q4h × 4. How many g of the medication should the patient receive? _____

47. You are to give 1 g of Keflex. You have capsules labeled 500 mg. How many capsules should you give? _____

48. A patient is to receive digitoxin 0.6 mg, PO Stat. You have available digitoxin tablets of the following sizes: 0.05 mg, 0.1 mg, 0.15 mg, and 0.2 mg. Which one(s) should you give? _____

49. You are to compute the amount of drug for a patient who weighs 154 pounds. Five milligrams

are to be given for every kilogram of body weight. How many milligrams of the drug will be needed? _____ This equals how many grams? _____

50. As a patient can have 10 mg Compazine q6h prn for nausea. In the past 3 days she has required five doses. How many grams of Compazine has she received so far? _____

51. A patient is to receive Valium 10 mg, tid. The available tablets are labeled 5 mg and 2 mg. What should you give for each dose? _____

52. The patient is to receive six Telepaque tablets 10 hours prior to her gallbladder x-ray. Each tablet contains 500 mg. How many grams should she receive? _____ How many milligrams is the total dose? _____

53. A patient is to have 100 mg of Colace qd. Capsules are available in 50 mg and 100 mg. What should you give for each dose? _____ How many grams should be received each day? ___

54. A 19-inch, 7-pound infant is _____ cm long and _____ Kg heavy.

55. A 33-pound child is to receive 0.1 mg of a medication per Kg of body weight. How much of the drug will be needed? _____

56. A 220-pound man is to receive 5 mg of a medication per Kg of body weight. How much of the drug will be needed? _____

57. A patient is to receive 2 g of Velosef per day in equal divided doses q6h. How many mg should he receive at each administration? _____

Answers to Metric System Practice Problems

1.	1000	20.	0.001	39.	5
2.	1000	21.	0.0002	40.	31.5
3.	0.5	22.	200	41.	.001
4.	10	23.	0.0005	42.	6
5.	50	24.	0.00004	43.	2 tab
6.	2	25.	40	44.	4 tab
7.	0.5	26.	1200	45.	12 cap
8.	0.05	27.	0.4	46.	1 g
9.	1000	28.	500	47.	2 cap
10.	500	29.	0.05	48.	Three 0.2-mg tab
11.	300	30.	2	49.	350 mg .35 g
12.	15	31.	20	50.	.05 g
13.	8	32.	5	51.	Two 5-mg tab
14.	0.008	33.	110	52.	3 g 3000 mg
15.	0.01	34.	4	53.	100 mg .1 g
16.	0.005	35.	8.8	54.	48.3 cm 3.18 Kg
17.	0.015	36.	22.7	55.	1.5 mg
18.	0.03	37.	54.5	56.	500 mg
19.	0.06	38.	0.05	57.	500 mg

UNIT TWO

CALCULATION OF FRACTIONAL DOSAGE

Medications are manufactured in various forms: solid drug forms such as tablets and capsules and liquid forms such as aqueous solutions (syrups), aqueous suspensions (mixtures and emulsions), and alcohol solutions (elixirs, tinctures, and extracts). When computing the correct dosage of a medication, the nurse is determining the amount of the drug form needed to administer the volume of drug ordered.

1. The drug vehicles most frequently administered by the nurse are the solid forms, tablets and capsules, and the liquid forms, measured by the volume of ml. The drug vehicle is the drug form in which the medication is available. In order to determine the amount of medication to administer, the nurse must first identify the amount or concentration of drug carried by the drug's _____.

form *or* vehicle

2. Colace is available in 100-mg capsules. The basic vehicle for Colace is one capsule, each of which carries 100 mg of the drug. The amount of drug is usually obvious when the solid forms of capsules and tablets are the vehicles. However, many people have difficulty perceiving that the liquid vehicle measure of ml should be treated in the same fashion as the solid drug vehicles. Demerol is available in 30-cc vials, with each ml of volume containing 50 mg of Demerol. The base vehicle unit in this situation is _____ ml instead of one capsule or tablet.

1

3. In the above example the 300-cc vial would contain _____ mg of Demerol, with each ml containing _____ mg.

1500
50

4. What are the drug *vehicles* for the following medication orders?
   a. Aspirin 650 mg qid (aspirin is available in 325-mg tablets supplied in boxes of 100 tablets) _____

1 tablet

   b. Morphine 10 mg IM q4h prn (morphine is available in 10 mg/ml in a 30-cc vial) _____

1 ml

5. For the above aspirin example, how much aspirin does the entire box of 100 tablets contain? _____ How many tablets of aspirin are needed to deliver the 650-mg dose? _____

32,500 mg
2

6. For the above morphine example, how much morphine is contained

22

300 mg
1

in the 30-cc vial? _____ How many ml are needed to deliver the 10-mg dose? _____

7. In these two examples, the arithmetic involved in computing the doses to be administered is fairly easy. However, in more complex problems the proportion formula can be used to compute the amount of the base vehicle to be administered for a given drug order. For example:

Drug order: Erythromycin .5 g q6h
Drug form available: 250-mg capsules
Proportion: (see pp. 3 and 4 for explanation of proportion problems)

$$\text{(drug unit)} \atop \text{(vehicle)} \quad \frac{250 \text{ mg}}{1 \text{ cap}} :: \frac{500 \text{ mg}}{? \text{ cap}} \text{ (drug order)}$$
$$250x = 500$$
$$x = 2$$

2

How many capsules are needed for each dose? _____
Note that the same units of measure must be used in working proportion problems. Therefore in this calculation both of the drug amounts must be stated in either mg or g.

8. Although these next problems can be solved easily with simple division, use the proportion formula to practice its application. Determine the number of vehicles to administer for each of the following doses:

   a. Drug order: Aldomet 500 mg tid
      Form available: 250-mg capsules

$$\frac{250 \text{ mg}}{1 \text{ cap}} :: \frac{500 \text{ mg}}{? \text{ cap}}$$

2

   Each dose = _____ caps

   b. Drug order: Diabinese 125 mg qd
      Form available: 250-mg *scored* tablets

½

   Each dose = _____ tablet

   c. Drug order: Orinase 750 mg bid
      Form available: 500-mg scored tablets

1½

   Each dose = _____ tablets

9. To compute the correct volume of a liquid medication to be administered, use the volume measure of ml as the drug vehicle. If Demerol 75 mg is ordered to be given Stat and the 30-cc vial is labeled "Demerol 50 mg/ml," what volume should be given? _____

1.5 ml

$$\frac{50 \text{ mg}}{1 \text{ ml}} :: \frac{75 \text{ mg}}{? \text{ ml}}$$

10. Work the following problems:
    a. Drug order: Compazine 10 mg IM q6h prn for nausea
       Form available: 5 mg/ml in 10-ml vials

       Each dose = _____ ml
    b. Drug order: Teldrin syrup 4 mg tid
       Form available: 2 mg/5 ml in 120-ml bottles

       Each dose = _____ ml
    c. Drug order: Benadryl Elixir 25 mg tid
       Form available: 12.5 mg/5 ml in 120-ml bottles

       Each dose = _____ ml
11. For the preceding Benadryl order, how many doses does each 120-

    ml bottle of the elixir contain? _____ How much Ben-
    adryl does a full bottle contain? _____
12. Some parenteral medications do not store well when suspended in
    solution. After a few hours, days, or weeks, the drug may begin to
    deteriorate. Also, some drugs need to be refrigerated when sus-
    pended in solution. Therefore, such drugs are stored in a powder
    form. When the drug is to be injected, it is first dissolved or sus-

    pended in a _____.
13. When a drug in powder form is to be administered parenterally, it

    must first be _____ in a sterile water, saline, or
    dextrose solution.
14. Unless specifically stated on the label, the amount of solution used
    to dissolve the sterile powder depends only on the convenience of
    the amount to be used. You may determine how much sterile water
    to use to dissolve the powdered drug unless a required amount is

    specifically stated on the _____.
15. A guideline to follow is that an injection of under 2 ml will cause
    only slight discomfort. If more than 5 ml of solution is injected into
    one site, tissue damage may occur because of pressure. Therefore,
    when it is possible, dissolve powdered drugs in an amount of so-
    lution that will allow one dose to be contained in approximately

    _____ ml of solution.
16. Usually a vial label indicates the minimum amount of solution nec-
    essary to dissolve the powder in the vial as well as what solution
    should be used. When a vial is a multiple-dose vial (one that con-
    tains more than one dose), try to use an amount of solution to dis-
    solve the drug that will allow each dose to be contained in approx-

    imately _____ ml or less.
17. In multiple-dose vials, the powder to be dissolved often adds to the
    final total volume of liquid in the vial. When this is the case, the
    label indicates the amount of solution to use to dissolve the powder
    and the total volume this will achieve. This total volume will in-

clude the powder volume factor. For example, if a vial contains 1 g of Cefazolin powder and you are to give 500 mg IM, you must first dissolve the powder in sterile water. The label states, "Dissolve powder in 2.5 ml. Total volume will equal 3 ml." This vial would then contain _____ mg/3 ml.

1000

18. How much Cefazolin would be required for the 500-mg dose? _____ ml

1.5

$$\frac{1000 \text{ mg}}{3 \text{ ml}} :: \frac{500}{? \text{ ml}}$$

19. A vial contains 250 mg of ampicillin powder. The label indicates that 2 ml of sterile water or normal saline are necessary to dissolve the powder. When the powder is dissolved, the volume will equal 2.5 ml. You are to give 100 mg q6h. Each dose will require _____ ml.

1

20. Most medications are standardized by the *United States Pharmacopeia* (USP) according to their active chemical ingredients and can therefore be measured with the usual weight or volume measurements. However, some medications in the antibiotic, hormone, and vitamin groups are standardized by the effects they have on animals. The USP unit is used to measure these drugs. Also, some minerals are measured by milliequivalents (mEq). A milliequivalent is the valence or charge of the drug times the milligram weight divided by the molecular weight.

$$mEq = valence \times \frac{mg \text{ wt}}{mol \text{ wt}}$$

However, regardless of whether the drug is measured in mEq, units (U), or mg, the same formula is used to determine the amount of the vehicle to use. For example, if you are to give 150,000 U of penicillin and the vial contains 300,000 U/ml, how many milliliters should you give? _____

.5 ml

$$\frac{150,000 \text{ U}}{? \text{ ml}} :: \frac{300,000 \text{ U}}{1 \text{ ml}}$$

21. Work the following problems:
    a. You are to add potassium chloride 30 mEq to an intravenous solution. The 20-cc vial label reads KCl 40 mEq/20 ml. How much should you use? _____

15 ml

$$\frac{40 \text{ mEq}}{20 \text{ ml}} :: \frac{30 \text{ mEq}}{? \text{ ml}}$$

2 ml

5 ml

units

100

insulin

concentration

U100

b. You are to add 20,000 U of heparin to a liter of IV solution. The form available is a 4-ml vial with 10,000 U per ml. How much should you use? _____

c. You are to add 10 mEq of KCL to 1000 cc of D5 .45 NS IV solution. The 10-cc vial has a label that reads KCL 20 mEq/10 ml. How much should you add to the IV solution? _____

22. Insulin is used in replacement therapy for diabetes. The drug forms in which insulin are available have been standardized. In the past, insulin was available in the three drug concentrations of 40 U, 80 U, and 100 U per ml. As of March 24, 1980, the Food and Drug Administration of the United States stopped certifying insulin preparations with the concentration of 80 U per ml. Currently insulin is available in 10-cc vials containing 40 U/ml or 100 U/ml as well as 20-cc vials containing 500 U/ml. The nurse must still read the labels on the insulin vials to determine not only which type of insulin they contain, but also how many _____ are in each milliliter.

23. Insulin syringes are designated to measure insulin by its unit concentration. When insulin preparations containing a concentration of 40 U/ml are used, a U40 scale syringe is needed to measure the correct dose. When insulin with a 100 U/ml concentration is used, a U _____ scale syringe is needed to measure the correct dose.

24. The measurement of insulin is the only situation in dosage calculation that does not require identifying the amount of drug form to administer. This medication is measured according to its drug unit amount using a matching-unit syringe. When administering insulin, always use an _____ syringe calibrated with the unit concentration of the insulin preparation to be used.

25. When administering insulin, make sure that the scale on the syringe used to measure the insulin corresponds to the _____ of the insulin being used.

26. Note the U100 scale syringe below. When full, this syringe holds only 1 ml of insulin. The only concentration of insulin that should be measured in this syringe is _____ insulin.

U100 scale

Insulin syringe

27. Although insulin preparations of 40 U and 500 U are available, most diabetics now use the 100 U/ml insulin concentration and many hospitals stock only the U100 concentration. When U100 insulin is used, a U _____ scale insulin syringe must be used for its measurement.

100

28. The use of the 100 U/ml concentration offers the advantage of reducing the volume needed to deliver a dose. If insulin with 40 U/ml is used to deliver a 40-U dose of insulin, _____ ml of this insulin will be needed. However, if insulin with 100 U/ml is used to deliver the same 40-U dose, only _____ ml will be needed.

1

.4

$$\frac{100\ U}{1\ ml} :: \frac{40\ U}{x} \qquad \begin{aligned} 100x &= 40 \\ x &= .4\ ml \end{aligned}$$

29. As can be seen, U100 insulin concentrations have the advantage over lower insulin concentrations of delivering a given dose in a *(smaller? larger?)* volume.

smaller

30. A patient is taking a dose of 80 U of NPH insulin daily. His doctor has told him to use U100 insulin. How many units of the U100 insulin should he use for his daily dose? _____

80 U

31. To measure insulin, always use the dosage amount rather than the drug-form volume. To ensure this type of measurement, always measure U100 insulin with a _____ scale insulin syringe.

U100

32. Identify the insulin measurements to be used for the following orders:

a. The patient is to receive 10 U of regular insulin and 30 U NPH insulin qd. U100 insulin is available for both types of insulin. Using a U_____ scale syringe, _____ U of regular insulin and _____ U of NPH insulin should be administered.

100; 10
30

b. Order: 5 U regular and 40 U Lente insulin q am. U100 insulin is available. Using a U100 insulin syringe, _____ U of regular and _____ U of Lente should be administered.

5
40

Fractional Dosage Practice Problems

1. You have 15 mg/ml of morphine sulfate available. The order is for 10 mg to be given. How much of the solution should you administer? _____

2. The codeine sulfate tablets are labeled 30 mg. You are to give 60 mg. How many tablets should you administer? _____

3. Tylenol tablets are labeled 0.325 g. How many tablets are needed for a dose of 650 mg? _____

4. You are to give Demerol 75 mg. The label on the vial reads Demerol 1 ml = 50 mg. How much of the solution should be used? _____

5. You are to give penicillin 400,000 U. The label reads penicillin 300,000 U/ml. How much should you use? _____

6. The vial of powdered material is labeled Staphcillin 1 g. The directions say to add 1.5 ml of sterile saline. The solution will then equal 2 ml. How much of the solution should you give if the order is Staphcillin 500 mg IM? _____

7. How many 10-mg doses of morphine can be given from a 10-ml vial that contains morphine 15 mg/ml? _____

8. You are to obtain 2 g of magnesium sulfate from a solution labeled 25 g/100 ml. How many milliliters do you need? _____

9. You are to administer potassium chloride 60 mEq intravenously. The label on the vial reads potassium chloride 20 ml = 40 mEq. How much should you use? _____

10. You are to give Fer-In-Sol 300 mg qd. Form available: 50-ml dropper bottle with 125 mg/ml. How much should you give per dose? _____

11. Drug order: Talwin 75 mg q3–4h prn. Form available: 50-mg scored tablets. How much should be given per dose? _____

12. Drug order: Indocin 50 mg tid. Form available: 25-mg capsules. How much should be given per dose? _____

13. Drug order: Mycostatin 1,000,000 U tid. Form available: 500,000-U tabs. How much should be given per dose? _____

14. Povan is to be given for pinworms: 5 mg/Kg of body weight. The patient weighs 30 Kg. Form available: oral suspension with 50 mg/5 ml. How much should be given per dose? _____

15. Drug order: Pro-Banthine 15 mg ac and 30 mg hs. Form available: 15-mg tab. How many tablets should be given each day? _____

16. You are to add 3000 U of heparin to a liter of IV solution. Form available: 10-ml vial of 1000 U/ml. How much should you use? _____

17. You are to add 15 mEq KCl to a liter of IV solution. Form available: 20-ml vial containing 40 mEq. How much should you use? _____

Drug order: Lente insulin 20 U bid.
Concentration available: Lente insulin U100.
Syringe available: U100.

18. How many units of this insulin should be given? _____

Drug order: NPH insulin 30 U qd of U100 NPH.

19. Which insulin concentration should be used?_____
20. Which syringe scale must be used to measure this dose? _____
21. How many units of the above should be given? _____

Drug order: Regular insulin 60 U qd.
Concentration available: U40, U100.

22. Which concentration will deliver 60 U via the smallest volume? _____
23. If U100 concentration is used, which insulin syringe should be used? _____
24. How many units of U100 should be given for this dose? _____
25. Drug order: Staphcillin 1 g IM q6h. Form available: 1-g vial of powder to be dissolved in 1.5 ml sterile water. Total volume = 2 cc. How many ml should be given per dose? _____
26. Drug order: Penicillin G potassium 500,000 U q6h. Form available: 1,000,000-U vial of powder. If powder is dissolved in 3.6 ml of sterile water, there will be 250,000 U/ml. How many ml should be given per dose? _____
27. Drug order: Ancef 500 mg IM tid. Form available: 1-g vial of powder. The label states that the powder should be diluted in 2.5 cc of sterile water for IM injections. Total volume will equal 3 cc. How many ml should be given per dose? _____
28. Drug order: Cefoxitin 1 g IV qid. Form available: 2-g vial of powder. The label states that the powder should be diluted in 20 cc of sterile water for IV use. Total volume equals 21 cc. How many ml should be given per dose? _____
29. Drug order: Tobramycin 60 mg IV tid. Form available: 80 mg in a 2-cc vial. How many ml should be given per dose? _____
30. Drug order: Amikacin at a level of 15 mg/kg/day to be given in 3 equally divided doses. The patient weighs 110 pounds. How much amikacin should be given per day? _____ per dose? _____ If amikacin is available in 2-cc vials containing 500 mg each, how many ml are needed per dose? _____

Answers to Fractional Dosage Practice Problems

1. 0.66 ml
2. 2 tabs
3. 2 tabs
4. 1.5 ml
5. 1.3 ml
6. 1 ml
7. 15 doses
8. 8 ml
9. 30 ml
10. 2.4 ml

11. 1.5 tabs
12. 2 caps
13. 2 tabs
14. 15 ml
15. 5 tabs
16. 3 ml
17. 7.5 ml
18. 20
19. U100
20. U100

21. 30
22. U100
23. U100
24. 60
25. 2 ml
26. 2 ml
27. 1.5 ml
28. 10.5 ml
29. 1.5 ml
30. 750 mg
    250 mg
    1 ml

UNIT THREE   APOTHECARIES' SYSTEM

In the recent past, a second system of weighing and measuring drugs has been used in the United States: the apothecaries' system. Currently, most drugs are measured using the metric system. However, because some institutions and physicians still make use of some of the apothecaries' measures, it is necessary for a nurse to be aware of what the apothecaries' system includes.

1. The apothecaries' system is of ancient derivation and deals only with units of weight and volume. The metric system, as you recall, deals with measures of length, weight, and volume, but the apothecaries' system deals only with the measurement of _____ and _____.

    weight
    volume

2. In the apothecaries' system, the smallest unit of weight is the *grain*. This unit of weight is so called because in ancient times a millet grain was used to balance the material being weighed. The smallest unit of weight in the apothecaries' system is the _____.

    grain

3. As you can see by the example of the millet grain, the apothecaries' unit used for measuring very small quantities is the _____.

    grain

4. The weight unit of grain is abbreviated gr. Always use gr to avoid confusing the grain with the gram, which is abbreviated g. The abbreviation for grain is _____.

    gr

5. The gram is about 15 times larger than a grain; confusing the two could be very serious. The abbreviation for grain is _____. The abbreviation for gram is _____.

    gr
    g

6. The next largest unit of weight in the apothecaries' system is the scruple, and it takes 20 gr to equal it in weight. However, this measure is seldom used. The smallest unit of weight in the apothecaries' system is the _____, and the next largest is the scruple.

    grain

7. The dram, the next largest unit of weight after the scruple, is equal to 60 gr. The word *dram* originated from the Greek drachma, a silver coin that was supposed to weigh approximate-

dram

gr

3

grain; gr

60

480 gr
8
60

3

3; 8

3

Eight
60; 480

3 x

ly the same as the dram. The unit of weight that equals 60 gr is the _____.

8. As you remember, the grain is abbreviated _____. However, a special symbol, instead of an abbreviation, is used for the dram. The written symbol that represents the dram looks like this: 3. It looks something like a sideways V with a tail on it. There are 60 gr in a _____ (use written symbol).

9. The smallest unit of weight in the apothecaries' system is the _____, and it takes 60 _____ to make a dram. All quantities less than a dram are expressed in grains.

10. The grain is the apothecaries' dry weight measure most frequently used by the nurse. Although the pharmacist may use the dry dram weight, which equals _____ gr, the nurse almost never administers an amount of drug this large.

11. The pharmacist also uses the ounce unit of weight. The ounce is equal to 8 3. If there are 8 3 in an ounce and 60 gr in 1 3, how many grains are in an ounce? _____

12. An ounce is equal to 480 gr because an ounce equals _____ 3, and 1 3 equals _____ gr (8 × 60 = 480).

13. The ounce also has its own written symbol, which is very similar to the symbol for the dram. The symbol for the dram is _____, whereas the symbol for the ounce is 3. Note that the difference between the two symbols is that the ounce symbol has one more zigzag on the top.

14. The ounce is the larger unit of weight of the two measures; its symbol also has more zigzags. The symbol for the ounce is _____, and it takes _____ 3 to equal the ounce in weight.

15. The largest apothecaries' dry weight unit is the pound (lb). This pound equals 12 ounces. What is the symbol for ounces? _____

16. Although there is an apothecaries' pound, it is almost never used. The most frequently used weights of the apothecaries' system are the grain, dram, and ounce. _____ drams equal an ounce, _____ gr equal a dram, and _____ gr equal an ounce.

17. In the metric system, only Arabic numerals are used to express quantities. In the apothecaries' system, however, whenever symbols or abbreviations are used, the quantity is expressed in small Roman numerals following the symbol or abbreviation. For example 3 grains is gr iii, and 10 ounces is 3 x. How should 10 drams be written? _____

18. A dot or a line is placed over the numeral for one to avoid confu-

ʒ iv

sion with the Roman numeral L, meaning 50. If 4 grains is written gr iv, how is 4 drams written? _____

19. This rule holds true for quantities under 40 (xxxx) units. Quantities over 40 are usually expressed in Arabic numerals in front of the apothecaries' symbol, for example, 480 gr. Also, when the quantity is a fraction or a number containing a fraction, it is expressed in Arabic numerals following the unit (for example, gr ¼ or gr ⅙). If

ʒ viii

gr ⅙

60 gr

7 ounces is written ℥ vii, how is 8 drams written? _____
If ¼ grain is written gr ¼, how is ⅙ grain written? _____
How is 60 grains written? _____

20. The one exception to this rule is the symbol expressing the fraction ½. The symbol ss is used to express the fraction ½. The symbol ss is derived from the word *semi,* meaning one half. If 7½ grains is

gr viss

written gr viiss, how is 6½ grains written? _____

21. In the apothecaries' system, the measurement of liquid volume closely parallels the apothecaries' units of dry weight. The smallest unit of apothecaries' weight, the _____, equals the smallest

grain

unit of volume, which is the minim (♍).

22. One dram is equivalent to 60 gr. Because the measures of weight and volume parallel each other, and because a fluidram equals ʒ i,

60

a fluidram should contain _____ ♍.

60; 60

23. It takes _____ gr to equal ʒ i, and it takes _____ ♍ to equal a fluidram (fʒ).

24. Note that an *f* is included in the written symbol for fluidram. It refers to the fluid measure rather than the dry measure.

♍

f ʒ

f ℥

The abbreviation of minim is _____.
The symbol for fluidram is _____.
The symbol for fluidounce is _____.

25. Fill in the proper equivalents.

60

viii

60

viii

fʒ i = _____ ♍
f℥ i = fʒ _____
ʒ i = _____ gr
℥ i = ʒ _____

26. The small medicine glass used in hospitals (p. 34) is usually fluidounce size. The nurse frequently administers amounts of liquid medication as large as fluidrams or a fluidounce. However, when drugs are administered in their dry weight form, the nurse seldom administers units larger than a *(gr? ʒ? ℥?).*

27. Frequently, volumes much larger than fluidounces are used. Most of these measures are commonly used in the home, so they should be familiar. For example, 2 pints (pt or O) equal 1 quart (qt), and 4 quarts equal 1 gallon (C). These are quantities in which milk and

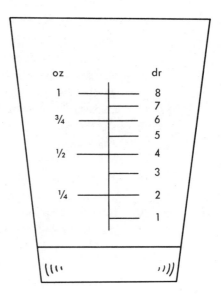

other fluids are commonly sold. If you bought qt i of milk, you
would also have pt _____. If you bought C i of milk, you
would have pt _____ or qt _____.

ii

viii; iv

28. One equivalent you might not be familiar with is that it takes $f\!\!\mathfrak{z}$ xvi
to equal pt i. It takes twice as many fluidounces to equal a pint as
it takes fluidrams to equal a fluidounce; therefore, $f\mathfrak{z}$ _____
equals $f\!\!\mathfrak{z}$ i, and $f\!\!\mathfrak{z}$ _____ equals pt i.

viii

xvi

29. At this point the parallel of the dry weight and liquid volume measurements breaks down. It takes only $\mathfrak{z}$ xii of dry weight to equal
1 lb, but it takes $f\!\!\mathfrak{z}$ _____ to equal pt i of liquid volume.

xvi

30. Fill in the proper equivalents.

viii
60
xvi
viii
60
iv
ii

$\mathfrak{z}$ i = $\mathfrak{z}$ _____
$f\!\mathfrak{z}$ i = _____ ${\rm m}$
pt i = $f\!\!\mathfrak{z}$ _____
$f\!\!\mathfrak{z}$ i = $f\!\mathfrak{z}$ _____
$\mathfrak{z}$ i = _____ gr
C i = qt _____
qt i = pt _____

31. In some textbooks and in hospital usage, the symbol $\mathfrak{z}$ is used for
the symbol $f\!\mathfrak{z}$. However, you can tell from the property of the
material whether the symbol refers to dry weight or liquid volume.
You may also find the symbol $\mathfrak{z}$ used interchangeably for the symbol _____.

$f\!\mathfrak{z}$

32. As with the metric system, when you are computing drug dosages

form *or* vehicle

using the apothecaries' system, you can use the proportion method to determine the amount of the drug's _____ to administer.

33. Work the following problems:

a. Drug order: Aspirin gr x
Available form: gr v tabs

2 tab

How many should be given? _____

$$\frac{gr\ v}{1\ tab} :: \frac{gr\ x}{?}$$

b. Drug order: nitroglycerin gr $\frac{1}{150}$
Available form: gr $\frac{1}{300}$ tab

2 tab

How many tab should be given? _____

$$\frac{gr\ \frac{1}{150}}{?} :: \frac{gr\ \frac{1}{300}}{1\ tab}$$

If review of fractions is needed, see p. 2.

Review of Apothecaries' System Equivalents

Weight:	60 grains (gr)	= 1 dram (ℨ)
	8 drams or 480 grains	= 1 ounce (℥)
	12 ounces	= 1 pound (lb)

Volume:	60 minims (♏)	= 1 fluidram (fℨ)
	8 fluidrams or 480 minims	= 1 fluidounce (f℥)
	16 fluidounces	= 1 pint (pt or O)
	2 pints	= 1 quart (qt)
	4 quarts	= 1 gallon (C)

Apothecaries' System
Practice Problems

1. $f\!\!\!3$ i = $\mathfrak{m}$ _____
2. $f\!\!\!3$ iii = $\mathfrak{m}$ _____
3. $f\!\!\!\xi$ xvi = qt _____
4. $f\!\!\!\xi$ xvi = pt _____
5. 60 $\mathfrak{m}$ = $f\!\!\!3$ _____
6. 3 viii = ξ _____
7. ξ ss = 3 _____
8. 3 iii = gr _____
9. ξ viii = gr _____
10. ξ viss = gr _____
11. $f\!\!\!3$ iv = $\mathfrak{m}$ _____

12. $f\!\!\!\xi$ viii = pt _____
13. $f\!\!\!\xi$ xxxii = qt _____
14. $f\!\!\!\xi$ iv = $\mathfrak{m}$ _____
15. pt iii = $f\!\!\!\xi$ _____
16. pt ss = $\mathfrak{m}$ _____
17. gr xv = 3 _____
18. gr xxx = 3 _____
19. gr xx = 3 _____
20. $f\!\!\!3$ viii = $f\!\!\!\xi$ _____
21. gr xxiv = ξ _____
22. $f\!\!\!3$ ii = $f\!\!\!\xi$ _____

23. You are to give gr iss of Seconal. You have capsules containing gr ¾. How many capsules should you give? _____

24. You are to give gr x of ferrous gluconate. You have gr v tablets. How many should you give? _____

25. You are to administer elixir of terpin hydrate $f\!\!\!3$ i. How many doses will a ξ iv bottle contain? _____

26. How much morphine sulfate would be required to make up $f\!\!\!\xi$ ii of a solution if every $\mathfrak{m}$ xx of the solution is to contain gr ¼? _____

27. Drug order: Digoxin gr ¹⁄₃₀₀ qd. Available form: tablets gr ¹⁄₆₀₀. How many should be given? _____

28. Drug order: Atropine gr ¹⁄₂₀₀ SQ. Available form: gr ¹⁄₁₅₀/ml. How much should be given? _____

29. Drug order: Colchicine gr ¹⁄₅₀ q2h up to 16 times or until pain subsides. Tablets gr ¹⁄₁₀₀ are available. If 10 doses are needed to reduce the pain, how many tablets would the patient receive? _____

How many grains of colchicine will have been ingested? _____

Answers to Apothecaries' System Practice Problems

1. 60
2. 1440
3. ss
4. i
5. i
6. i
7. iv
8. 180
9. 3840
10. 3120
11. 240
12. ss
13. i
14. 1920
15. 48
16. 3840
17. ¼
18. ss
19. ⅓
20. i
21. ¹⁄₂₀
22. ¼
23. 2 cap
24. 2 tabs
25. 32 doses
26. gr xii
27. 2 tabs
28. 0.75 ml
29. 20; gr ⅕

UNIT FOUR

CONVERSION OF APPROXIMATE EQUIVALENTS

Although efforts are being made to establish the metric system as the standard for drug measurement, the nurse may still encounter drug orders written in the apothecaries' system although the packaged drug is labeled using the metric system. When this occurs, the nurse must convert the drug measurement into the metric system. In the past, the frequent interchange between the two measurement systems made it important for a nurse to have memorized the ratios used to convert measures between the systems. However, because drugs are now so infrequently ordered in the apothecaries' system, it is difficult for a nurse to remember the conversion rules and ratios. Given the current level of use, it appears important now that a nurse understand the principles of conversion and be familiar with reading a conversion table.

1. The apothecaries' system deals only with measures of weight and volume, so the only measures that can be converted from the apothecaries' system to the metric system are those dealing with units of

weight; volume

_____ and _____.

2. When converting a measurement from system to another, you should first identify whether you are working with units of weight

weight

or volume. The gram and grain are both measures of _____.

3. Identify which of the following measure units of weight. (Place a check in the correct blanks.)

	a.	ℳ
b	b.	gr
c	c.	Kg
	d.	ml
e	e.	g
f	f.	ʒ
	g.	fʒ
h	h.	mg
	i.	cc
	j.	qt

4. An apothecaries' unit of weight can be converted only to a unit of metric _____.

5. When one system is converted to the other, the exact equivalents frequently include fractional parts of units. For example: the exact equivalent of 1 gram is 15.432 grains. For easier handling, the *United States Pharmacopeia* established a standard of approximate equivalents that rounds these numbers off to more manageable figures. Although 1 g exactly equals 15.432 gr, the acceptable approximate equivalent is 1 g = gr xv. This rounded off approximation is limited to a 10% change. That is, the number to which the equivalent is rounded does not differ by more than 10% of the exact equivalent. For example, 10% of 15.432 is 1.5432. Therefore, the convenient, easily manipulated number of 15 does not require a change from 15.432 of greater than 10%. The approximate equivalent of 1 g is gr _____.

6. Because each grain equals $\frac{1}{15}$ of a gram, the ratio of grams to grains in the standard of approximate equivalents is 1 : _____.

The following are the approximate *weight* equivalents standardized by the *United States Pharmacopeia:*

$$1 \text{ Kg} = 2.2 \text{ lbs}$$
$$30 \text{ g} = ʒ \text{ i}$$
$$4 \text{ g} = ʒ \text{ i}$$
$$0.06 \text{ g} = \text{gr i}$$
$$1 \text{ g} = \text{gr xv}$$

gr xv	= 1 g	= 1000 mg
gr x	= 0.6 g	= 600 mg
gr viiss	= 0.5 g	= 500 mg
gr v	= 0.3 g	= 300 mg
gr iii	= 0.2 g	= 200 mg
gr iss	= 0.1 g	= 100 mg
gr i	= 0.06 g	= 60 mg
gr ¾	= 0.05 g	= 50 mg
gr ss	= 0.03 g	= 30 mg
gr ¼	= 0.015 g	= 15 mg
gr ⅙	= 0.01 g	= 10 mg
gr ⅛	= 0.008 g	= 8 mg
gr 1/12	= 0.005 g	= 5 mg
gr 1/15	= 0.004 g	= 4 mg
gr 1/20	= 0.0032 g	= 3 mg
gr 1/30	= 0.0022 g	= 2 mg
gr 1/60	= 0.001 g	= 1 mg
gr 1/100	= 0.0006 g	= 0.6 mg

$$\text{gr } \tfrac{1}{120} = 0.0005 \text{ g} = \quad 0.5 \text{ mg}$$
$$\text{gr } \tfrac{1}{150} = 0.0004 \text{ g} = \quad 0.4 \text{ mg}$$
$$\text{gr } \tfrac{1}{200} = 0.0003 \text{ g} = \quad 0.3 \text{ mg}$$
$$\text{gr } \tfrac{1}{300} = 0.0002 \text{ g} = \quad 0.2 \text{ mg}$$
$$\text{gr } \tfrac{1}{600} = 0.0001 \quad = \quad 0.1 \text{ mg}$$

7. Using this table of weight equivalents, identify the apothecaries' units that are equivalent to the following metric units.

8 mg = gr _____

.008 g = gr _____

30 mg = gr _____

1 g = gr _____

.2 mg = gr _____

.0006 g = gr _____

8. Now, using the table, identify the metric units equivalent to the following apothecaries' units.

gr viiss = _____ g or _____ mg

gr iss = _____ g or _____ mg

gr $\tfrac{1}{120}$ = _____ g or _____ mg

gr v = _____ g or _____ mg

gr $\tfrac{1}{15}$ = _____ g or _____ mg

gr $\tfrac{1}{30}$ = _____ g or _____ mg

9. When the apothecaries' unit to be converted is gr i or smaller, it is usually more convenient to use the mg approximate equivalent.

1 g = gr _____; 1 gr = _____ mg

10. The above approximations provide base ratios that can be used in proportion calculations to convert g and mg to gr. For example, because 1 g = gr xv, the number of g in gr xxx can be determined by using a proportion calculation.

$$\frac{1 \text{ g}}{\text{gr xv}} :: \frac{? \text{ g}}{\text{gr xxx}}$$

gr xxx = _____ g

11. Use a proportion calculation to determine how many mg = gr i.

$$\frac{1 \text{ g}}{\text{gr xv}} :: \frac{? \text{ g}}{\text{gr i}}$$

gr i = _____ g or _____ mg

Left margin answers:

⅛
⅛
ss
xv
1/300
1/100

.5; 500
.1; 100
.0005; .5
.3; 300
.004; 4
.0022; 2

xv; 60

2

.06; 60

12. When calculating proportions, remember that the ratio units must remain the same. That is, if the base ratio measurement units are g to gr, the answer must be stated in these measurement units. If the base ratio is g to gr, an mg equivalent can be obtained only by converting the g answer to mg. This is done by multiplying the grams by _____ or moving the decimal 3 places to the right.

13. If the apothecaries' amount to be converted is less than gr i, the base ratio of gr i = 60 mg can be used to determine the approximate equivalent in the metric measure. For example, if gr i = 60 mg, how many mg does gr ss equal?

$$\frac{\text{gr i}}{60 \text{ mg}} :: \frac{\text{gr ss}}{? \text{ mg}}$$

$$\text{gr ss} = \text{_____ mg}$$

14. The two base ratios that can be used to convert gr to g and gr to mg are gr xv = _____ g and gr i = _____ mg. However, because apothecaries' weight conversions are so infrequently required, it is safer for the nurse to refer to a conversion table than to trust to memory.

15. Because most pharmaceutical preparations are labeled by metric measure, the usual conversion problem the nurse faces is the conversion of a drug order written in the apothecaries' system to the _____ system, by which the medication is labeled.

16. Drug order: Nitroglycerin gr 1/150 prn
Form available: Nitroglycerin .4-mg tab
  a. Convert the dosage:
    gr 1/150 = _____ mg
  b. The number of .4-mg tablets needed to deliver the gr 1/150 dose is _____.

17. Drug order: Digitoxin gr 1/300 qd
Form available: Digitoxin .1-mg tab
  a. Convert the dosage:
    gr 1/300 = _____ mg
  b. How many tablets are needed? _____

18. Drug order: Morphine gr 1/8 q4h prn
Form available: 20-cc vial of morphine, 10 mg/ml
  a. gr 1/8 = _____ mg
  b. How much morphine should be given per dose? _____

19. Drug order: Codeine gr ss q4h prn

Form available: 30-mg tab

30   **a.** gr ss = _____ mg

1   **b.** Tablets required for dosage? _____

20. The primary need the nurse will have in conversion of weight measures from the apothecaries' system to the metric system is from gr

xv; 60   to g or mg. 1 g = gr _____; gr i _____ mg. Although the other weight measures of ʒ and ℥ can also be converted to the metric system, the nurse does not usually have to do this because the apothecaries' weight the nurse usually works with is

gr   _____. The equivalent weights of the ʒ and ℥ can be found in the review section at the end of this unit.

21. Conversions in the volume measurements are more common than dry weight measure conversions. The volume measures of the

fʒ; f℥   apothecaries' system are the $\mathfrak{m}$, _____, and _____.

22. In the apothecaries' system, the units of volume and weight parallel each other. Remember from Unit Three that it takes the same number of minims to equal a fluidram as it does grains to equal a dram.

60; 60   gr _____ = ʒ i; $\mathfrak{m}$ _____ = fʒ i.

viii   **23.** Also, it takes ʒ viii to equal an ounce and fʒ _____ to equal f℥ i.

24. The fact that the weights and volumes parallel each other is very helpful, because you can use the same ratios with the volume units as you did with the weight units. The ratio between the grain and

15; 1   gram is _____ : _____.

25. Likewise, the ratio between the minim and the cubic centimeter or

15   milliliter is _____ : 1. (Remember that these two units, the cubic centimeter and the milliliter, are equal.)

26. Using the 15 : 1 ratio between the minim and the milliliter, work the following problems:

150   **a.** 10 ml = $\mathfrak{m}$ _____

$$\frac{1 \text{ ml}}{\mathfrak{m} \text{ xv}} :: \frac{10 \text{ ml}}{\mathfrak{m} \text{ ?}}$$

60   **b.** 4 ml = $\mathfrak{m}$ _____

3   **c.** .2 ml = $\mathfrak{m}$ _____

27. If it takes $\mathfrak{m}$ xv to fill a cubic centimeter and $\mathfrak{m}$ 60 to equal to

4   fluidram, then it takes _____ ml to equal a fluidram.

28. Using the ratio of 4 ml : fʒ i, do the following problems:

     a. fʒ ii = ? ml

43

$$\frac{f\mathfrak{Z}\ i}{4\ ml} :: \frac{f\mathfrak{Z}\ ii}{?\ ml}$$

$f\mathfrak{Z}$ ii = _____ ml

b. $f\mathfrak{Z}$ 250 = _____ ml
c. $f\mathfrak{Z}$ v = _____ ml
d. 6 ml = $f\mathfrak{Z}$ _____
e. 16 ml = $f\mathfrak{Z}$ _____

29. If _____ ml = $f\mathfrak{Z}$ i and $f\mathfrak{Z}$ _____ = $f\mathfrak{z}$ i, then it would seem that there should be _____ ml in a fluidounce.

30. However, the approximation that has been established for the fluidounce is 30 ml. Most medicine glasses are an ounce size. Note the use of both the dram and ml scale on the medicine glass. Because

$f\mathfrak{z}$ i = 30 ml, then $f\mathfrak{z}$ ss = _____ ml.

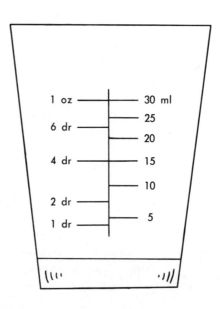

31. Although $f\mathfrak{Z}$ iv would seem to equal 16 ml, because $f\mathfrak{Z}$ i = 4 ml,

$f\mathfrak{Z}$ iv has been approximated to 15 ml. $f\mathfrak{z}$ i = _____ ml, $f\mathfrak{z}$ ss = _____ ml, and $f\mathfrak{Z}$ iv = _____ ml.

32. Because 30 ml = $f\mathfrak{z}$ i, the ratio between $f\mathfrak{z}$ and ml is _____ : _____.

33. Do the following problems.
a. $f\mathfrak{z}$ vi = ? ml

$$\frac{f\mathfrak{z}\ i}{30\ ml} :: \frac{f\mathfrak{z}\ vi}{?\ ml}$$

$f\mathfrak{z}$ vi = _____ ml

120
15

ii

ss
vi

minim
xv; 30; 4

1000; 1000
1000

500
2
500

1
500
4
1000
30
15
15

i
xv
xv
30
4

b. $f℥$ iv = _____ ml
c. $f℥$ ss = _____ ml
d. 60 ml = $f℥$?

$$\frac{f℥\ i}{30\ ml} :: \frac{?\,f℥}{60\ ml} \qquad 60\ ml = f℥\ \underline{\hspace{2cm}}$$

e. 15 ml = $f℥$ _____
f. 180 ml = $f℥$ _____

34. All of the units of volume in the apothecaries' system are larger than the milliliter except the *(minim? dram? ounce?)*.

35. ♏ _____ = 1 ml; _____ ml = $f℥$ i; _____ ml = $f℥$ i.

36. There are two more units of volume in the apothecaries' system of which you should know the metric equivalents. The first one is the quart, which is approximately equal to the same volume as the liter. The liter equals _____ ml or _____ cc. Therefore, the quart also equals _____ ml.

37. If the quart equals 1000 ml, ½ quart or a pint would equal _____ ml.

38. There are _____ pt in a quart; so a pint would equal _____ ml if a quart equals 1000 ml.

39. Fill in the proper equivalents.
_____ ml = ♏ xv
_____ ml = pt i
_____ ml = $f℥$ i
_____ ml = qt i
_____ ml = $f℥$ i
_____ ml = $f℥$ ss
_____ ml = $f℥$ iv

40. Fill in the proper equivalents.
gr _____ = 60 mg
gr _____ = 1 g
♏ _____ = 1 ml
$f℥$ i = _____ ml
$f℥$ i = _____ ml

Review of Conversion Equivalents

Volume:
$$1 \text{ ml} = \mathfrak{m} \text{ xv}$$
$$1 \text{ cc} = \mathfrak{m} \text{ xv}$$
$$0.06 \text{ ml} = \mathfrak{m} \text{ i}$$
$$4 \text{ ml} = f\mathfrak{z} \text{ i}$$
$$30 \text{ ml} = f\mathfrak{z} \text{ i}$$
$$500 \text{ ml} = \text{pt i}$$
$$1000 \text{ ml} = \text{qt i}$$

Weight:
$$1 \text{ Kg} = 2.2 \text{ lb}$$
$$30 \text{ g} = \mathfrak{z} \text{ i}$$
$$4 \text{ g} = \mathfrak{z} \text{ i}$$
$$0.06 \text{ g} = \text{gr i}$$
$$1 \text{ g} = \text{gr xv}$$

gr xv	= 1 g	= 1000 mg
gr x	= 0.6 g	= 600 mg
gr viiss	= 0.5 g	= 500 mg
gr v	= 0.3 g	= 300 mg
gr iii	= 0.2 g	= 200 mg
gr iss	= 0.1 g	= 100 mg
gr i	= 0.06 g	= 60 mg
gr ¾	= 0.05 g	= 50 mg
gr ss	= 0.03 g	= 30 mg
gr ¼	= 0.015 g	= 15 mg
gr ⅙	= 0.01 g	= 10 mg
gr ⅛	= 0.008 g	= 8 mg
gr 1/12	= 0.005 g	= 5 mg
gr 1/15	= 0.004 g	= 4 mg
gr 1/20	= 0.0032 g	= 3 mg
gr 1/30	= 0.0022 g	= 2 mg
gr 1/60	= 0.001 g	= 1 mg
gr 1/100	= 0.0006 g	= 0.6 mg
gr 1/120	= 0.0005 g	= 0.5 mg
gr 1/150	= 0.0004 g	= 0.4 mg
gr 1/200	= 0.0003 g	= 0.3 mg
gr 1/300	= 0.0002 g	= 0.2 mg
gr 1/600	= 0.0001 g	= 0.1 mg

Conversion Practice Problems

Use the conversion table to determine weight equivalents.

1. ℳ xxx = _____ml
2. pt i = _____ml
3. qt i = _____ml
4. ʄ℥ ss = _____ml
5. gr viiss = _____g
6. gr ss = _____mg
7. gr ¹⁄₁₅₀ = _____mg
8. gr ¾ = _____g
9. 4 g = _____gr
10. 4 ml = ʄ℥ _____

11. gr ¹⁄₃₀₀ = _____ mg
12. gr ¼ = _____ mg
13. 30 ml = ʄ℥ _____
14. 50 mg = gr _____
15. 5 mg = gr _____
16. 0.001 g = gr _____
17. 0.015 g = gr _____
18. 0.3 g = gr _____
19. 0.6 g = gr _____

20. You are to give Seconal gr iss. You have 50-mg capsules. How many should you give? _____

21. Drug order: Aspirin gr x q4h PO prn. (When doses are as large as gr v, medications are now being packaged in metric units, which are closer to the exact equivalents than are the standardized approximate equivalents. The exact equivalent of gr v = .333 g. The dosage being packaged now is 325-mg. Although aspirin used to be packaged in 300-mg tablets, it is now packaged in 325-mg tablets.) If you have 325-mg tablets available, how many should you give for this drug order per dose? _____

22. You are to give ferrous gluconate gr v. You have 325-mg tablets. How many should you give? _____

23. You are to give morphine gr ⅙. You have a vial with 10 mg/ml. How many ml should you give? _____

24. You are to give milk of magnesia 30 ml. How many fluidounces should you give? _____

25. You are to give chloral hydrate gr xv. You have .5-g capsules on hand. How many should you use? _____

26. You are to give Aludrox ℥ ii. How many milliliters should you give? _____

27. You are to give aspirin gr x, qid × 7 days. The pharmacy has 325-mg and 650-mg tablets available. Which kind of tablet and how many should you order? _____

28. You are to give morphine gr ¼. You have a vial with 10 mg/ml. How many ml should you give? _____

29. The patient is to receive Lugol's solution ℳ v, tid. How many ml must you order from the pharmacy for the solution to last 8 days? _____

30. You are to give Maalox 15 ml, q2h. If you have a ʄ℥ xvi bottle, how many doses will it contain? _____

31. You are to give 30 mg of codeine. The vial contains gr ss/ml. How many ml should you give? _____

32. You are to give gr ½₀₀ of atropine. The vial contains .4 mg/ml. You should give _____ ml.

33. You are to give Compazine gr ⅙. The vial contains 5 mg/ml. How much should you give? _____

34. You are to give phenobarbital gr ss. You have 15-mg, 30-mg, and 60-mg tablets on hand. What should you give? _____

Answers to Conversion Practice Problems

1. 2
2. 500
3. 1000
4. 15
5. 0.5
6. 30
7. 0.4
8. 0.05
9. 60
10. i
11. 0.2
12. 15

13. i
14. ¾
15. $\frac{1}{12}$
16. $\frac{1}{60}$
17. ¼
18. v
19. x
20. 2 caps
21. 2 tabs
22. 1 tab
23. 1 ml

24. *ʒ* i
25. 2 caps
26. 8 ml
27. 28 650-mg tabs
28. 1.5 ml
29. 8 ml
30. 32 doses
31. 1 ml
32. .75
33. 2 ml
34. One 30-mg tab

HOUSEHOLD MEASURES

1. A graduated container for accurate measurement may not be available in the home and some household articles may have to be used to measure approximately the amount required. Household measures deal only with the measurement of liquid drugs. However, they are not accurate and should be avoided in the administration of drugs in the hospital, because they are gross measures and only _____ the amount required.

approximate

2. One of the most common household measures used is the unit of the drop. A drop is approximately equivalent to the minim in volume. Because the drop (gtt) is not always equal to the minim, medicine is not usually measured in gtt unless so ordered by the doctor. The approximate equivalent of the drop is the _____.

minim

3. Because there are $\mathfrak{m}$ xv in a ml, there also are approximately _____ gtt in a ml.

15

4. The drop is most frequently used in the hospital in the calculation of the infusion rate of an IV solution. By counting the number of drops per minute that fall from the bottle of fluid into the IV tubing, you can calculate the number of ml being infused per minute. If each ml of IV solution equals 15 gtt, and 15 gtt fall every minute, then the solution would be infusing at the rate of _____ cc/ minute.

1

5. At this rate of infusion, how long should it take for 60 cc of solution to infuse? _____

1 hour

6. Because nurses use this measure so frequently to monitor IV flow rates, Unit Six is devoted to the calculation and monitoring of IV infusion rates. The household measure the _____ (gtt) is used to calculate IV flow rates.

drop

7. Another household measuring unit commonly used is the teaspoon (t). The teaspoon is the approximate equivalent of the fluidram.

4     $f\mathfrak{Z}$ i = _____ ml

i   1 t = $f\mathfrak{Z}$ _____

4   1 t = _____ ml

1

8. On a medicine glass, you will find that $f\mathfrak{Z}$ i, 4 ml, and _____ t are all equal measures.

i; 4

9. One teaspoonful is equal to $\mathfrak{Z}$ _____ and _____ ml.

viii; 8

10. If $\mathfrak{Z}$ i = $\mathfrak{Z}$ _____, then $\mathfrak{Z}$ i = _____ t.

11. Every fluidounce also contains 2 tablespoonfuls (T).

4

If $f\mathfrak{Z}$ i = 8 t, then 1 T = _____ t.

12. The teaspoon used to determine this equivalent was the common teaspoon, not the cooking teaspoon. The common teaspoon =

4

_____ ml, but the cooking teaspoon = 5 ml.

13. Because the use of metric measures has become prevalent, drug companies are preparing liquid medications with the usual pre-scribed amount of the drug carried in the unit vehicle of 5 ml rather than the measure of a $\mathfrak{Z}$. If the medication ordered carries its drug amount in the unit vehicle of 5 ml, the common teaspoon should not be used for the drug's measurement. The cooking teaspoon is

5

more accurate because it contains _____ ml.

4

14. The teaspoon measures found on medicine glasses equal _____ ml, but most liquid medications are now often carried in the unit

5

vehicle of _____ ml.

cooking

15. The equivalent measure of 5 ml is the _____ teaspoon. Many drug companies package such a teaspoon or a small medicine glass with liquid medications so that 5 ml can be conveniently and accurately measured in the home.

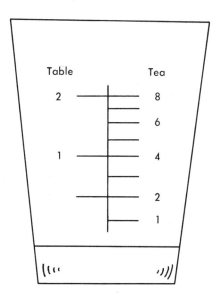

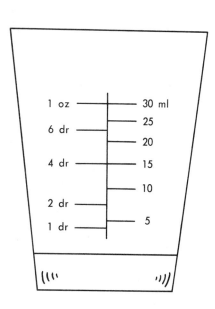

16. Give the standard approximate equivalents for the following:

1   _____ gtt = ℥ i

30   _____ ml = $f℥$ i

15   _____ gtt = 1 ml

2   _____ T = $f℥$ i

viii $f℥$ _____ = $f℥$ i

2   _____ T = 30 ml

1   _____ t = $f℥$ i

4   common t = _____ ml

5   cooking t = _____ ml

17. The three main areas in which the nurse makes use of household equivalents are as follows:

    a. Calculating IV fluid flow

liquid   **b.** Measuring _____ drugs in the home

    c. Calculating the amount of fluid a patient drinks

18. When a nurse keeps a record of the amount of fluid a patient drinks, the teacupfuls and glassfuls of liquid drunk are counted. A teacup-

180   ful usually holds $f℥$ vi; so, brimful, a teacup should hold _____ ml, because $f℥$ i = 30 ml and 30 × 6 = 180.

19. Because the teacup is usually not filled to the brim, its capacity is

150   usually calculated as $f℥$ v, which equals _____ ml.

20. An ℥ viii glass is the size of drinking glass commonly used in the hospital. A glass of this size, full to the brim, would hold 240 ml of fluid, because 8 × 30 ml equal 240 ml. However, usually these glasses are not completely full, so they are calculated to hold only 200 ml. This figure is rounded off in this manner for easier com-

200   putation. One glass is equal to _____ ml.

150   **21.** A teacup is equal to $f℥$ v, or _____ ml, and a glass is equal

200   to _____ ml.

1000   **22.** If a patient drank 5 glasses, he would have drunk _____ ml of fluid.

200; 150   **23.** A glass equals _____ ml, and a teacup equals _____ ml. If a patient drank 4 glasses of water and 3 teacups of coffee,

1250   his liquid intake would total _____ ml.

It must be realized, of course, that these are only gross approximations. If it is essential that the measurement of a patient's intake be very accurate, this method would not be appropriate.

24. Fill in the following:

2   _____ T = $f℥$ i

15   _____ gtt = 1 ml

4   _____ ml = 1 common t

150   _____ ml = 1 teacup

30   _____ ml = 2 T

200   _____ ml = 1 glass

1   _____ gtt = ♏ i

4   _____ ml = ʄȝ i

5   _____ ml = 1 cooking t

Review of Household Equivalents

60 drops (gtt)   = 1 teaspoonful (t)
4 teaspoonfuls   = 1 tablespoonful (T)
2 tablespoonfuls = fluidounce
6 fluidounces   = 1 teacupful
8 fluidounces   = 1 glassful

Household	Apothecaries'	Metric
1 drop	= 1 minim	= 0.06 ml
1 teaspoonful	= 1 fluidram	= 4 ml
1 cooking teaspoon =		5 ml
1 tablespoonful	= 4 fluidrams	= 15 ml
2 tablespoonfuls	= 1 fluidounce	= 30 ml
1 teacupful	= 6 fluidounces	= 180 ml
1 glassful	= 8 fluidounces	= 240 ml
1 teacup	= 5 fluidounces	= 150 ml
1 glass	= 6⅔ fluidounces	= 200 ml

Household Measures Practice Problems

1. 1 teacup = _____ml
2. 1 glass = _____ml
3. 1 t = ƒȝ _____
4. 30 ml = _____T
5. ƒȝ i = _____t
6. ƒȝ i = _____T

7. ℥ i = _____gtt
8. 1 T = _____ml
9. 15 gtt = _____ml
10. 5 ml = _____t
11. 4 glasses = _____ml
12. 15 ml = _____T

13. You are instructing a mother about how to give her child 5 ml of cough syrup at home. What household measure can she use? _____

14. If a patient is to take ƒȝ i of milk of magnesia at home, what household measure can he use? _____

15. It is recorded on a patient's intake slip that he has drunk 1000 ml of fluid. How many glasses does this equal? _____

16. If a patient has drunk 2 teacups and 3 glasses of fluid, how many milliliters of fluid has he consumed? _____

17. Drug order: 2½ T of 10% KCL bid. How many ml should be administered per dose? _____ per day? _____

18. If a 10% KCL solution contains 40 mEq of KCL/30 ml, how much KCL is contained in 2½ T? _____

19. Drug order: Metamucil 1 T bid. How many ml should be administered per dose? _____

20. Drug order: 2 T of potassium gluconate bid. Elixir is available in 6.7 mEq/5 ml. How many ml are needed per dose? _____ How many mEq should be received per dose? _____ per day? _____

Answers to Household Measures Practice Problems

1. 150
2. 200
3. i
4. 2
5. 1
6. 2
7. 1

8. 15
9. 1
10. 1 cooking
11. 800
12. 1
13. 1 cooking t
14. 2 T

15. 5 glasses
16. 900 ml
17. 37.5 ml
    75 ml
18. 50 mEq
19. 15 ml
20. 30 ml
    40.2 mEq
    80.4 mEq

CALCULATION OF IV FLOW RATES

The household measure the drop (gtt) is most frequently used in the hospital in the calculation of the infusion rate of an IV solution. By counting the number of drops that fall each minute from the bottle or bag of IV fluid into the IV tubing's drip chamber, you can calculate the number of ml being infused per minute.

1. As you recall from Unit Five, 1 gtt = ℳi and ℳ xv = 1 ml. Therefore, the approximate household equivalent of 1 ml = _____ gtt.

   15

2. The eye of the dropper greatly influences the actual number of gtt required to move 1 cc of fluid into the IV drip chamber. The label on the IV tubing box will indicate the dropper capacity of the specific tubing being used. The most frequent dropper capacities are 10 gtt/ml, 15 gtt/ml, 20 gtt/ml, and 60 gtt/ml. Although the usually accepted equivalent is _____ gtt/ml, always check the IV tubing box for the stated dropper capacity.

   15

3. To calculate the gtt of IV solution that should be administered per minute, you need to calculate the amount of fluid to be delivered per hour, the number of drops to be administered per hour, and then the drops per minute. To calculate the ml that should be delivered in 1 hour, divide the total fluid volume ordered by the number of _____ over which the fluid is to infuse.

   hours

4. The second step in IV flow rate calculation is to determine how many drops should be administered in 1 hour. Do this by multiplying the dropper rate by the hour volume. The usual dropper capacities are 10 gtt/ml, _____ gtt/ml, 20 gtt/ml, and 60 gtt/ml.

   15

5. If you are to administer 100 ml of IV fluid in an hour and you have an IV tubing with a 10 gtt/ml capacity, you should deliver _____ gtt/hour. (Dropper rate × hour volume = 10 × 100)

   1000

6. To calculate the number of drops per minute, you divide the number of drops per hour by _____.

   60

7. Do the following problem: The doctor has written an order for 1000 ml of 5% glucose to be administered in 8 hours. How many drops

must be administered per minute? (Round fraction of drops to the nearest whole even number.)

a. How many milliliters must be administered per hour?

8; 125

    1000 ml ÷ _____ hr = _____ ml per hour

The dropper rate is 15 gtt/ml.

1875

b. 125 ml × 15 gtts = _____ gtt/hour

1875; 32

c. _____ gtt ÷ 60 minutes = _____ gtt per minute

8. If you are to administer 500 cc of D$_5$W (5% glucose) intravenously within 5 hours,

100

a. How many ml should infuse per hour? _____

b. If the dropper capacity is 10 gtt/cc, how many gtt does 100 ml

1000

    equal? _____

16

c. Therefore, _____ gtt should flow per minute to administer 100 ml/hour. (1000 ÷ 60)

9. Try one more problem: 250 ml of 5% glucose must be administered in 2 hours (dropper rate 15 gtt/ml).

125

a. _____ ml per hour

1875

b. _____ gtt/hour

c. If you administer 1875 gtt per hour, you then should administer

32

    _____ gtt per minute in order to have 250 ml completely administered in 2 hours.

10. If you are to administer 250 cc of .9% NaCl solution in an 8-hour period and the dropper capacity is 60 gtt/cc, how many drops per

32

    minute should be administered? _____

10; 15

11. The usual dropper capacities are _____ gtt/ml, _____

60

gtt/ml, 20 gtt/ml, and _____ gtt/ml.

12. The 10-, 15-, and 20-gtt/ml capacity drippers are referred to as macrodrop administration sets. The 60-gtt/ml set is referred to as a minidrop set. Because there are fewer drops/cc delivered by the

larger

macrodrop sets, they deliver *(larger? smaller?)* drops.

13. In order for an IV solution to infuse, the hydrostatic pressure in the IV system must be greater than that in the venous system. If it is not, the flow of solution will cease owing to blood flowing into the IV tubing or blood-clot formation in the lumen of the IV needle.

slowly

Macrodrop sets will drip drops of solution more *(slowly? rapidly?)* into the drip chamber than will minidrop sets.

14. When a macrodripper is used to deliver IV solution at a rate of under 60 cc/hour, the drip rate is so slow that the hydrostatic pressure may fall to a level that stops the IV flow in the intervals between the drips. For this reason when fluids are administered at a rate of under 50 cc/hour, you should use a minidrop set that delivers

60

    _____ gtt/ml.

15. The more frequent dripping of a minidrop set will maintain a more constant level of hydrostatic pressure in the IV system. Some hospitals, to provide an extra margin of clot prevention, set the flow rate for minidrop set use at under 80 cc/hour. A minidrop set delivers _____ gtt/ml.

16. On the other hand, when larger volumes of fluid are to be administered, the minidrip sets may be unable to deliver larger volumes owing to the small drop size. Usually a macrodrop set is needed when volumes of over 125 cc/hour are to be administered. Macrodrop sets include drippers with capacitites of _____ gtt/ml, _____ gtt/ml, and _____ gtt/ml.

17. One of the factors to consider when calculating IV fluid flow rates is the type of drip capacity that should be used. If under 60 cc/hour will be delivered, use a _____ drop set. If more than 125 cc/hour will be delivered, use a _____ drop set.

18. IV order: 500 cc .9% NaCl solution over 10 hours.
    a. How many ml should be administered in 1 hour? _____
    b. Which dripper should be used? _____
    c. How many drops should be delivered per hour? _____
       (50 × 60)
    d. How many drops should be delivered per minute? _____

19. If you had used a 10-gtt/ml dripper in the above situation, how many drops per minute would be needed? _____ (Round fractions of drops to the nearest whole even number.)

20. You are to administer 3000 cc of NS (normal saline or .9 NaCl solution) over the next 24 hours.
    a. How many ml per hour should be administered? _____
    b. Should a 60- or 10-gtt/ml dripper be used? _____
    c. How many drops per minute are needed? _____
    (Round out your answer.)

21. IV order: Bottle #1 1000 cc LR (Lactated Ringer's solution)
                Bottle #2 1000 cc NS
                Bottle #3 1000 cc D₅W
    All three are to run in over 24 hours.
    Using a 15-gtt/ml dripper, how many drops are needed per minute to deliver this volume? _____

22. 500 cc D₅W/LR is to run over 8 hours per minidrip. How many drops are needed per minute? _____

23. A patient is to receive 20 cc/hour of IV solution. How many drops per minute are needed? _____ You of course would use a _____ drop set.

24. Notice in the last two problems the number of drops to be received per minute is the same number as the number of cc to be adminis-

tered per hour. This is because you both multiplied and divided the number of cc/hr by _____.

$$20 \text{ cc/hour} \times \frac{60 \text{ gtt/ml}}{60 \text{ minutes/hour}}$$

When a minidrop set is used, the gtt delivered per minute is the same as the cc of solution delivered per hour because the number of gtt/ml and minutes/hour cancel each other out of the equation.

25. The above example identifies a shortcut for calculating IV flow rates. The ratio between the gtt/ml and minutes/hour can be used to calculate the flow rate by multiplying that ratio by the cc to be delivered per hour. If the drip rate is 60 gtt/ml, and 40 cc/hour of solution will be administered, the gtt/minute should be.

$$40 \text{ cc/hour} \times \frac{60 \text{ gtt/ml}}{60 \text{ minutes/hour}} =$$

40

_____ gtt/minute

26. If the drip rate is 10 gtt/ml, the ratio between 10 gtt/ml and 60 minutes/hour is 1:6.

Therefore, the cc/hour would be divided by 6. If 100 cc will be administered per hour, how many drops per minute are needed?

$$100 \text{ cc/hour} \times \frac{10 \text{ gtt/ml}}{60 \text{ minutes/hour}} =$$

16

$$100 \times \frac{1}{6} = \frac{100}{6} = \text{_____ gtt/minute}$$

27. If, in the same problem, the drip rate were 15 gtt/ml, what would the drip rate per minute be? The ratio between 15 gtt/ml and 60 minutes/hour is 1:4. Therefore, the cc/hour would be divided by

4

_____ .

$$100 \text{ cc/hour} \times \frac{15 \text{ gtt/ml}}{60 \text{ minutes/hour}} =$$

25

$$100 \times \frac{1}{4} = \frac{100}{4} = \text{_____ gtt/minute}$$

28. If the drip rate in the same problem were 20 gtt/ml, what would the drip rate be per minute? The ratio between 20 gtt/ml and 60

minutes/hour is 1:3. Therefore, the cc/hour would be divided by

_____ .

$$100 \text{ cc/hour} \times \frac{20 \text{ gtt/ml}}{60 \text{ minutes/hour}} =$$

34

$$100 \times \tfrac{1}{3} = \tfrac{100}{3} = \underline{\hspace{2cm}} \text{ gtt/ml}$$

29. You are to administer 1000 cc NS in 5 hours using a 10-gtt/ml dripper. How many drops per minute are needed?

200

    a. How many cc/hour are needed? _____

    b. How many gtt/min?

$$200 \text{ cc/hour} \times \frac{10 \text{ gtt/ml}}{60 \text{ minutes/hour}} =$$

34

$$\tfrac{200}{6} = \underline{\hspace{2cm}} \text{ gtt/minute}$$

30. You are to administer 2000 cc D$_5$W in 10 hours using a 15-gtt/ml dripper. How many drops per minute are needed?

200

$$?/\text{hour} \times \frac{15 \text{ gtt/ml}}{60 \text{ minutes/hour}} =$$

$\tfrac{200}{4}$; 50

$$\tfrac{?}{?} = \underline{\hspace{2cm}} \text{ gtt/minute}$$

31. The use of this equation of

$$\text{volume/hour} \times \frac{\text{gtt/ml}}{\text{minutes/hour}}$$

will allow you to calculate IV flow rates using either the longer or shorter method of calculation. The three steps of the equation are

hour

1) calculate the cc to be delivered per _____ ; 2) calculate

hour

the drops to be delivered per _____ ; and 3) calculate the

minute

drops to be delivered per _____ .

32. You are to add 80 mg of tobramycin to 100 ml of D$_5$W and administer the IV medication using a secondary IV set. This is called administering a IV medication "piggyback" (or IVPB). If you are to run the medication over 30 minutes using a 10-gtt/ml dripper, how fast should the drop/minute rate be? You could either calculate the rate per hour by doubling the volume

$$200 \text{ ml/hour} \times \frac{10 \text{ gtt/ml}}{60 \text{ minutes/hour}} =$$

$$\frac{2000}{60} = 34 \text{ gtt/minute}$$

or calculate the rate for 30 minutes using the same formula

$$100 \text{ ml/}\frac{1}{2} \text{ hour} \times \frac{10 \text{ gtt/ml}}{30 \text{ minutes/}\frac{1}{2} \text{ hour}} =$$

30; 34

$$\frac{1000}{?} = \underline{\hspace{3cm}} \text{ gtt/minute}$$

or use the shortcut

$$100 \text{ ml/}\frac{1}{2} \text{ hour} \times \frac{10 \text{ gtt/ml}}{30 \text{ minutes/}\frac{1}{2} \text{ hour}} =$$

3; 34

$$\frac{100}{?} = \underline{\hspace{3cm}} \text{ gtt/minute}$$

33. Try another. Order: Ancef 1 g IV. You will dilute the medication in 50 cc D_5W and administer it using a 10-gtt/ml dripper over 15 minutes. How fast should the drop per minute rate be?

$$50 \text{ ml/}\frac{1}{4} \text{ hour} \times \frac{10 \text{ gtt/ml}}{15 \text{ minutes/}\frac{1}{4} \text{ hour}} =$$

15; 34

$$\frac{500}{?} = \underline{\hspace{3cm}} \text{ gtt/minute}$$

As you can see, the above equation for calculating IV fluid flow rate is composed of three steps:

a. Calculation of the cc volume to be delivered per a unit of time.

b. Calculation of the number of drops needed to deliver that volume in that time unit.

c. Calculation of the number of drops to be delivered in 1 minute of that time unit. Most often the time unit used is 1 hour because of its convenience, but the equation can be used to calculate the flow rate for any time unit.

$$\text{cc/time unit} \times \frac{\text{gtt/ml}}{\text{minute/time unit}} = \text{gtt/minute}$$

IV Flow Rate Practice Problems

1. If a doctor orders 1000 ml of 5% glucose IV fluid to be administered to a patient over the span of 6 hours, how many drops must be administered per minute using a 15-gtt/cc dropper? _____

2. IV order: 100 cc D_5W to be administered at 125 cc/hr. If a 10-gtt/cc dropper is used, how many gtt should be administered per minute? _____

3. IV order: 500 cc of .9% saline to be administered at 30 cc/hr. Using a 60-gtt/cc dropper, how many gtt should be administered per minute? _____

4. Order: 1000 cc LR to be followed by 2000 cc D_5W to run next 24 hours. What drop per minute rate is needed? You have a 10-gtt/ml tubing.

5. Order: 500 cc D_5W/NS at 100 cc/hour. What drop/minute rate is needed when a 15-gtt/ml tubing is used?

6. 500 cc D_5W/LR is to run over 8 hours. What drop/minute rate is needed? (What type of dripper do you need to use?)

7. 1000 cc LR is to run over 12 hours. What drop/minute rate is needed when using a minidrip?

8. Order: 1000 cc 2.5DW/.45NS to run 80 cc/hour. How many hours should this fluid run? What drop/minute rate is needed using a 20-gtt/ml dripper?

9. The doctor has ordered 1000 ml of IV fluid to run at 45 gtt/minute, using a 15 gtt/cc dropper. Approximately how long should the IV fluid run? _____

10. You are to administer an IV medication using the intravenous solution currently being administered at 100 cc/hour. The IV tubing has a metro set in it, which has a 10-gtt/ml drip rate. You let 50 cc of solution run into the metro set and add the medication to this volume. How long should it take for the medication to run in?

11. You are to give Ancef 1 g IV. You add this medication to a 50-cc bag of D_5W. Using a 10-gtt/ml secondary line you are to administer the medication within 10 minutes. How fast should the drop/minute rate be?

12. You are to administer Amikin 500 mg IVPB using a 15-gtt/ml secondary line. If the medication is diluted in 100 cc of D_5W, how fast should the drop/minute rate be to administer the medication in 40 minutes?

13. You are to give Decadron 6 mg IV. Decadron comes in a 5-ml vial with 4 mg/ml. You are to administer this medication in 50 cc of D_5W IVPB using a 10-gtt/ml secondary line. How many cc of Decadron should you add to the 50-cc secondary IV bag? What drop/minute rate is needed to administer the medication in 30 minutes?

14. Drug order: Cefoxitin 1 g tid. The vial available has 2 g of powder, which you are to reconstitute in 20 cc of sterile water. The reconstituted volume is 21 cc. You are to administer this mediation IVPB in 50 cc of D_5W using a 10-gtt/ml secondary line. How many cc of cefoxitin should be added to the 50-cc secondary bag? What should the drop/minute rate be to administer the medication within 20 minutes?

Answers to IV Flow Rate Practice Problems

1. 42 gtt
2. 20 gtt
3. 30 gtt
4. 20 gtt
5. 25 gtt
6. 62 gtt
   60 gtt/ml

7. 84 gtt
8. 12.5 hr
   26 gtt
9. 5.5 hours
10. 30 minutes
11. 50 gtt

12. 38 gtt
13. 1.25 cc
    16 gtt/minute
14. 10.5 cc
    30 gtt

SOLUTIONS FROM PURE DRUGS AND STOCK SOLUTIONS

1. Occasionally the nurse may have to prepare a drug solution from a pure drug or a stock solution. Pure drugs are substances in solid or liquid form that are 100% pure. Pure drugs are always considered

100 _____% pure unless otherwise stated. A stock solution is a relatively concentrated solution from which weaker solutions are made.

2. The easiest method of determining the amount of pure drug needed to make a solution is ratio-proportion. Whenever you work one of

100 these calculations, always consider a pure drug _____% pure unless otherwise stated.

3. The formula used to determine the amount of pure drug needed to make a solution is as follows:

$$\frac{\text{amount of drug}}{\text{amount of finished solution}} :: \frac{\% \text{ (of finished solution)}}{100\% \text{ (pure drug \%)}}$$

Notice that 100% is used because we are dealing with a

pure _____ drug.

4. To determine how much sodium perborate crystal is needed to make 250 ml of a 2% oral antiseptic solution, use the proportion formula:

5
$$\frac{x \text{ g}}{250 \text{ ml}} :: \frac{2\%}{100\%} \qquad 100x = 500 \qquad x = \text{_____} \text{ g}$$

5. For calculating the preparation of a solution, the weight and volume measures used must parallel each other and be in the same measurement system. The weight and volume measures in the previous

metric problem are both in the _____ system.

6. Because the kilogram is the parallel weight of the liter, the

gram _____ is the parallel weight of the milliliter.

7. If a g of a drug parallels a ml of solution, then a gr of a drug parallels a _____ of solution. To determine drugs weighed in mg, the proportion must be calculated using g to ml and the answer must be converted from g to mg.

8. Calculate how much salt is needed to make 500 ml of a .9% solution.

450; 4.5 g

$$\frac{x \text{ g}}{500 \text{ ml}} :: \frac{.9\%}{100\%} \qquad 100x = \text{_____} \qquad x = \text{_____}$$

9. Calculate how much glucose is needed to make 1 L of 5% glucose solution.

100; 5000

$$\frac{x \text{ g}}{1000 \text{ ml}} :: \frac{5\%}{100\%} \qquad \text{_____} \quad x = \text{_____}$$

50 g

$x = $ _____ of glucose

Always identify the vehicle weight or volume measure that is to be used.

10. When calculating a solution preparation, not only must you use the parallel weight and volume in the same _____ system, but also all solutions expressed in ratio or fractions must be translated into percents of solutions. For example: a ¼ or a 1:4 solution is a 25% solution. A fraction is changed to a percent by dividing the denominator into the numerator and multiplying by 100 (see pp. 2 and 3).

measuring

$$\text{¼} = 1:4 - \quad .25 = (.25 \times 100) \ 25\%$$
$$4\overline{)1.00}$$

11. Translate the following to percents.

5

.1

4

.2

10

%

1:20 solution = _____% solution

1:1000 solution = _____% solution

1:25 solution = _____% solution

1:500 solution = _____% solution

1:10 solution = _____% solution

12. Always change solutions expressed in fraction or ratio to _____ before calculating a solution preparation.

13. How much aluminum acetate is needed to make 500 ml of a 1:20 Burow's solution?

5

a. 1:20 = _____%

5

2500

25

b. $\dfrac{x \text{ g}}{500 \text{ ml}}$ :: $\dfrac{\%}{100\%}$

c. $100x = $ _____

$x = $ _____ g aluminum acetate

14. The amount of drug used to prepare a solution adds to the total volume of the solvent. The amount of volume contributed by a dry drug depends upon its individual structure. However, it is fairly easy to determine the volume that a liquid drug will add to the volume of the solvent. To determine the amount of water needed to make the finished solution, subtract the volume of the liquid drug from the amount of the finished solution. The volume of dry and

liquid

_____ drugs will contribute to the total volume of a finished solution.

15. The amount of volume added by a dry drug can be determined only by the structure of each individual drug; however, to determine the amount of water needed in the finished solution prepared with a

subtracted

liquid drug, the volume of the liquid drug is _____ from the volume of the finished solution.

16. For example: cresol is a liquid in its natural state. Determine how much cresol is needed to make a gallon of 2% saponated cresol solution:

   a. Calculate the volume of cresol needed.

80

$$\dfrac{x \text{ ml}}{4000 \text{ ml}} :: \dfrac{2\%}{100\%} \qquad x = \text{_____ ml cresol}$$

   b. Calculate the amount of water that is needed to produce a gallon of 2% saponated cresol solution.

   Finished solution = 4000 ml
   Cresol volume = 80 ml

   4000
   − 80

3920 ml
subtract
finished solution

   Water volume = _____

17. You must always _____ the amount of liquid drug from the volume of _____ to know how much water to add.

18. Whenever you prepare a solution from a stock solution rather than from a pure drug, the same principle of ratio and proportion is used. The only difference is that you are not working with 100% pure drug. A stock solution is a relatively concentrated solution from which weaker solutions are made. These stock solutions are not

pure

100% pure, so they cannot be considered _____ drugs.

19. The following formula is used to calculate the amount of stock solution that is needed to make a weaker solution.

$$\frac{\text{amount of drug}}{\text{amount of finished solution}} = \frac{\text{lesser }\%}{\text{greater }\%}$$

As you can see, this formula is much the same as the one used for

pure _____ drugs.

20. Complete the following: Prepare a quart of 4% formaldehyde fixative solution from a 37% stock solution.

108.1

$$\frac{x \text{ ml}}{1000 \text{ ml}} = \frac{4\%}{37\%} \qquad x = \text{_____ ml stock solution}$$

891.9

_____ ml water should be added.

21. Calculate the amount of 6% vinegar needed to prepare a gallon of .25% acetic acid.

166.6 ml

_____ vinegar

3833.4

_____ water

22. If you had a pint of 6% vinegar, how much .25% acetic acid solution could you make? _____

12,000 ml *or* 3 gallons

$$\frac{500 \text{ ml}}{x \text{ ml}} :: \frac{.25\%}{6\%}$$

How much water should you add to the pint of vinegar to obtain 3

11,500 ml

gallons of .25% acetic acid? _____

Pure Drugs and Stock Solutions Practice Problems

1. How much of a 1:20 solution of silver nitrate is needed to make a gallon of a 5% solution? _____

2. How much 1:20 Burow's solution is needed to make a liter of 1:40 solution? _____

3. How much 5.8% saline solution is needed to make 1 L of .9% solution? _____

4. How much glucose is contained in a liter of 5% glucose IV solution? _____

5. How much NaCl is contained in a liter of .9% NaCl IV solution? _____

6. The doctor has ordered 38 g of glucose to be given IV. How much 5% glucose solution should be used? _____

7. 1000 ml of a .45% NaCl and 2.5% dextrose IV solution will contain how much NaCl and dextrose? _____

8. A 50-cc vial contains 3.75 g of sodium bicarbonate. What is the percent of solution in this vial? _____

9. How much sodium bicarbonate is contained in 500 ml of a 5% IV solution? _____

10. How much water needs to be added to a liter of 75% isopropyl alcohol to change it to a 70% solution? _____

Answers to Pure Drugs and Stock Solutions Practice Problems

1. 400 ml
2. 500 ml
3. 155 ml
4. 50 g

5. 9 g
6. 760 ml
7. 4.5 g NaCl, 25 g dextrose

8. 7.5%
9. 25 g
10. 71.4 ml

CALCULATION OF INFANTS' AND CHILDREN'S DOSAGES

It is a nurse's responsibility to check that the drug dosage being administered to a patient is within the safe dosage range. However, two factors make meeting this responsibility more difficult with the pediatric patient:

1. Pharmaceutical companies supply most medications in standard adult dose strengths.
2. Because drug dosages are usually determined on the basis of body weight, and children vary in size, there are no convenient dosage ranges for children as there are for adults.

The most accurate way of determining whether a drug order for a child's dose is within a safe dosage range is to calculate the safe range on the basis of the suggested mg weight of the drug to be given per Kg of body weight of the child. This is usually determined for a 24-hour period. (mg/Kg body weight/24 hours)

For example, the drug order is methicillin 225 mg q6h. To determine if this dosage falls within the safe range, do the following:

1. Check a pediatric drug reference for the suggested dose per weight (methicillin sodium: 100 mg/Kg/24 hours: divide into 4–6 doses)*
2. Obtain the patient's weight (9 Kg)
3. Compare the drug order to the suggested dose

Order	*Suggested dose*
225 mg	100 mg
4/day	9 Kg
900 mg/24 hour	900 mg/24 hour

This comparison can also be done by dividing the child's weight into the amount of drug ordered/24 hours to see if it falls within or below the maximum range suggested in the pediatric drug references. In this example, the order was for 225 mg q6h or 900 mg/24 hours. The child weighed 9 Kg.

---

*Pediatric Dosage Handbook, American Pharmaceutical Association.

$$\frac{100 \text{ mg/Kg/24 hours}}{9 \text{ Kg)}900 \text{ mg}}$$

When the weight is divided into the amount of drug to be received, it is found that the child would receive a dosage that falls within the suggested pediatric dose of 100 mg/Kg/24 hours.

If the drug is not listed in the pediatric drug references, the following formulas are used, although the results are often inaccurate.

CHILDREN'S DOSAGES

Clark's rule:

$$\text{child's dose} = \frac{\text{weight of child (in pounds)}}{150 \text{ (average adult weight)}} \times \text{adult dose}$$

Cowling's rule:

$$\text{child's dose} = \frac{\text{age (in years on next birthday)}}{24} \times \text{adult dose}$$

Dilling's rule:

$$\text{child's dose} = \frac{\text{age (in years)}}{20} \times \text{adult dose}$$

Young's rule:

$$\text{child's dose} = \frac{\text{age of child (in years)}}{\text{age} + 12} \times \text{adult dose}$$

INFANTS' DOSAGES

Fried's rule:

$$\text{infant dose} = \frac{\text{age (in months)}}{150} \times \text{adult dose}$$

GENERAL ESTIMATE

½ year give $\frac{1}{24}$ adult dose
1 year give $\frac{1}{12}$ adult dose
2½ years give $\frac{1}{8}$ adult dose
5 years give $\frac{1}{4}$ adult dose
10 years give ½ adult dose
20 years give adult dose

Infants' and Children's Dosages Practice Problems

1. Drug order: Sudafed 10 mg PO qid. John is 9 months and weighs 8.6 Kg.
   a. If the usual child's dose is 5 mg/Kg/24 hours, how much can John receive to be within this range? _____
   b. Does his dose fall in this dose range? _____
   c. If Sudafed comes in a stock solution containing 30 mg/5 cc, how much should John receive per dose? _____
2. If John was changed to Ancef 50 mg IV qid and the usual children's dose was 25 mg/Kg/24 hours, does this dose fall safely within the suggested range? _____
   a. What dose will John receive in 24 hours? _____
   b. What dose level is suggested for this weight per 24 hours? _____
   c. Ancef is available in a vial containing 250 mg that, when diluted with 2 cc of sterile water, has a concentration of 125 mg/ml. What volume of Ancef should John receive per dose? _____
3. Susie, age 1, is to receive phenobarbital elixir 5 mg PO q8h. She weighs 5.7 Kg. If the usual dose is 1 mg to 6 mg/Kg/24 hours, how does Susie's dose compare?
   a. Is it safe? _____
   b. What dose is suggested per 24 hours for this weight? _____
   c. What dose is Susie to receive per 24 hours? _____
   d. The available ℥ viii bottle contains 20 mg/5 ml. How much should she receive per dose? _____
4. Jim is age 2½ and weighs 13 Kg. He is to receive 1 t qid of 125 mg/5 ml suspension of Keflex. The usual child's dose is 25 mg to 50 mg/Kg/24 hours.
   a. Is Jim's dose within the safe range? _____
   b. What amount of Keflex will he receive per 24 hours? _____
   c. What is the usual child's dose range for this weight for 24 hours? _____
   d. How many ml of Keflex should be received per dose? _____
5. Mary is age 1 and weighs 1720 g. She is receiving methicillin 35 mg IM q6h.
   a. If the usual child's dose of methicillin is 100 mg/Kg/24 hours, is Mary's dose safe? _____
   b. What dose is Mary receiving per 24 hours? _____
   c. What is the usual child's dose for this weight for 24 hours? _____
   d. How many ml of methicillin should Mary receive per dose if the 1-ml vial available contains 35 mg/0.25 cc? _____
6. Joe is age 7 and weighs 20 Kg. He is to receive the following as a preoperative medication:

Morphine 2 mg (usual child's dose = .05 mg to 0.1 mg/Kg/24 hours) and scopolamine .2 mg (usual child's dose = .02 mg/Kg/24 hours).

    a.   How much morphine can be given safely for a child this weight? _____

    b.   How much scopolamine can be given safely for a child this weight? _____

    c.   Are Joe's doses within safe limits? _____

    d.   The vials available contain morphine 10 mg/ml and scopolamine 0.4 mg/ml. How much of each medication should be given? _____

7. Margaret is age 13 years and weighs 38 Kg. She is to receive gentamicin 30 mg IV q8h. The usual child's dose is 3 mg/Kg/24 hours.

    a.   What dose/24 hours will she receive? _____

    b.   What is the usual suggested 24 hour dose for a child this weight? _____

    c.   Is Margaret's dose within the safe range? _____

    d.   Gentamicin is available in 2-cc vials containing 40 mg/ml. How much should she receive per dose? _____

    e.   If she were to receive this medication diluted in 50 cc of D_5W to run over a period of 40 minutes using a 10-gtt/ml tubing, what drop/minute rate would be needed? _____

8. Barb is 4 years and weighs 16 Kg. She is receiving erythromycin suspension 200 mg q6h. The usual child's dose is 30 mg to 50 mg/Kg/24 hours for mild infections and double that for severe infections.

    a.   What is the usual child's dose for this weight? _____

    b.   What daily dose is Barb receiving? _____

    c.   Is this within the safe range? _____

    d.   If this is available in pint bottles of 200 mg/5 ml, how much should she be receiving per dose? _____

    e.   How many doses of this size does the bottle contain? _____

    f.   How many days should it cover for Barb's dose? _____

Answers to Infants' and Children's Practice Problems

1. a. 43 mg/Kg/24 hours
   b. Yes (40 mg)
   c. 1.66 cc
2. Yes
   a. 200 mg
   b. 215 mg
   c. .4 cc
3. a. Yes
   b. 5.7 mg to 34.2 mg
   c. 15 mg
   d. 1.25 cc

4. a. Yes
   b. 500 mg
   c. 325 mg to 650 mg
   d. 5 ml
5. a. Yes
   b. 140 mg
   c. 172 mg
   d. .25 ml
6. a. 1 mg to 2 mg
   b. .4 mg
   c. Yes
   d. Morphine .2 ml
      Scopolamine .5 ml

7. a. 90 mg
   b. 114 mg
   c. Yes
   d. .75 cc
   e. 12 gtt/min
8. a. 480 mg to 1600 mg
   b. 800 mg
   c. Yes
   d. 5 ml
   e. 100
   f. 25

NOTES

NOTES

NOTES

NOTES

NOTES

NOTES

NOTES

NOTES

NOTES

NOTES